The MRCGP Study Book

GW00691687

The MRCGP Study Book

Second Edition

Eric Gambrill, MB BS, FRCGP, DRCOG
General Practitioner, Crawley, Sussex
Course Organiser, Crawley Vocational Training Scheme
Associate Adviser in General Practice, S. W. Thames Region
Examiner for the MRCGP

Alistair Moulds, MB, ChB, FRCGP, DRCOG
General Practitioner, Basildon, Essex
Course Organiser, Basildon Vocational Training Scheme
Organiser of MRCGP courses

John Fry, CBE, MD, FRCS, FRCGP
General Practitioner, Beckenham, Kent
Past Examiner for the MRCGP

David Brooks, MD, FRCGP, DRCOG
General Practitioner, Manchester
Associate Adviser in General Practice, Department of Postgraduate Medical Studies,
University of Manchester

Butterworths
London Boston
Singapore Sydney Toronto Wellington

Update–Siebert Publications
Guildford
Surrey

First edition published by Update Publications Ltd, 1981
Reprinted, 1982
Second edition, Butterworths/Update–Siebert, 1988

© **Eric Gambrill, Alistair Moulds, John Fry, David Brooks, 1988**

British Library Cataloguing in Publication Data

Gambrill, Eric
  The MRCGP study book.— 2nd ed.
  1. Great Britain. General practitioners.
  Professional education. Membership of the
  Royal College of General Practitioners'
  examinations
  I. Title   II. Moulds, A. J. (Alistair-John),
  1947–   III. Fry, John, 1922–
  610'.76

  ISBN 0-407-00432-7

Photoset by Butterworths Litho Preparation Department
Printed and bound in Great Britain at the University Press, Cambridge

Preface

Since the first edition of this book was published in 1981, a three-year vocational training for general practice has become mandatory for would-be principals. The exam has become well established and is recognised as an additional qualification by the General Medical Council. Now each year about 2000 trainees complete their training and most of them take the MRCGP examination. Why?

Apart from personal reasons, the principal reasons shared by nearly all candidates are first that the membership exam of the Royal College of General Practitioners is a test of the successfully completed training programme and second that possession of the MRCGP will help to achieve a good partnership appointment.

The MRCGP should not be a difficult examination to pass, yet there is a constant failure rate of about 1 in 3. This occurs not because the examiners are aiming to fail one third of the candidates but because the candidates fail themselves as a result of lack of preparation and application.

In this book we aim to help our readers to help themselves. It is not a text book, nor is it a 'crammer' on how to answer questions; rather it is a work book in which we invite the reader to take part in a plan of preparation for the examination that will take a few months. We trust this will assist prospective candidates with their problems and, indirectly, make the work of the examiners easier!

Eric Gambrill,
Alistair Moulds,
John Fry, and
David Brooks

Contents

Introduction

The decision to have an examination for membership of the Royal College of General Practitioners took some years of bitter debate. It was eventually introduced in 1965 when, on March 1, there were five candidates; all were successful.

The examination

The structure of the examination has evolved gradually since 1965 but is not in a set format. It consists of two stages: the first is a set of three papers, and this is followed some weeks later by two orals for those invited to attend. Note that there is no clinical part involving live 'patients', but there are many tests and questions on clinical subjects and methods.

The examination has been and is continually assessed to endeavour to make it a fair, valid and reliable test.

What is being tested?

The examination is broadly based on the content and job description as stated in the College's report on 'The Future General Practitioner – Learning and Teaching' (1972). This is not an easy book to read and its chief contribution has been to define five areas of learning and teaching:

1 Clinical practice – health and diseases.
2 Clinical practice – human development (at all ages).
3 Clinical practice – human behaviour.
4 Medicine and society.
5 The practice.

The examiners are out to test the candidate's knowledge, skills, attitudes and behaviour, and common sense in approaching the everyday and less usual situations and problems in general practice.

The format

The three written papers are:

1 Multiple choice questions (MCQs).
2 Modified essay questions (MEQs).
3 Practice topic questions (PTQs).

Approximately 80 per cent of all candidates will gain enough marks to be invited to the oral part.

With a final pass rate of around 70 per cent, it is evident that there will be failures at the orals. These parts are dealt with in detail in this book.

The examinees

The great majority of candidates at present are trainees who have completed, or almost completed, their vocational training programmes. Others are more senior NHS principals who seek to test themselves and some doctors from overseas.

The pass rates of the trainees are higher and reach 75–80 per cent.

1

The examiners

They are all practising general practitioners, almost all in the National Health Service (NHS). There are a few who are from university departments of general practice, but most are 'ordinary GPs' involved in vocational training. They read the journals, have practice libraries and are interested in recent trends in general practice. The questions that they will ask are those from ordinary general practices.

Why do candidates fail?

The chief reasons for failure are:

1 *Inadequate preparation* on the false assumption that participation in a vocational training is sufficient. It is not. We suggest a work plan as laid out on page 185.
2 *Inadequate knowledge* of basic facts on general practice (*see* pages 181–184) and lack of awareness of recent important publications.
3 *Poor examination techniques;* by involvement in the exercises that follow this should be corrected.
4 *Panic and nervousness* – remember that examiners are ordinary GPs, that usually there are no absolutely correct black-and-white answers and that your views will be respected if you make them clearly and cogently.
5 A poor basis of undergraduate education and language difficulties and, for overseas candidates, a lack of knowledge of the NHS – examiners should be told if a candidate comes from another health care system.

Practical points

1 The MRCGP examinations take place twice a year in mid-May and October–November (written papers), and July and December (orals). Results are announced immediately after completion of orals.
2 Closing dates for applications are about 8 weeks before the written papers.
3 There are three papers, MCQ, MEQ and PTQ, and orals with two sets of examiners.
4 Each part of the written examination is of equal value and accounts for 20 per cent of the total marks. It is not necessary for the candidate to pass each separate part in order to pass overall and an above average performance in one part can compensate for a poor performance in another part.
6 The marks from the three written papers are added together and averaged out. The candidates are placed into one of three groups: those *above the standardized mark*, about half of the candidates, who are automatically invited to the orals; those in the *weakest group*, one-fifth of the candidates, whose performance is so poor that they will have no chance of raising their marks and are not invited to the orals; the third *borderline group* (with average marks 42–50 per cent) who are currently invited to offer them a chance to do well in the orals.
6 It is important to make sure that you learn some of the *basic facts of general practice* and that you are familiar with *standard books and journals* to be able to refer to them in written and oral parts of the exam.

The Multiple Choice Question Paper or MCQ

Over the course of many years, MCQ papers have become established in nearly all branches of medicine as an effective and reliable means of assessing examinees' performance. They are mainly concerned with testing factual knowledge and recall and, if well constructed, are able to provide a reproducible assessment of knowledge which can accurately discriminate between candidates. The large number of candidates and the use of automatic marking means that the College MCQ is inherently reliable.

The MCQ paper is one of the five major parts of the MRCGP examination and, as such, is worth one-fifth of the total examination marks. Sixty questions, each of five parts, have to be answered in a total time of 2 hours. Each question is of the multiple true/false variety and comprises a 'stem' statement followed by five items or completions, e.g.

Erythema multiforme
('*Stem*')

   A Typical lesion is target shaped.
   B Recognized causes include sulphonamides.
   C Severe forms involve mucous membranes.
   D If patient is toxic, may be treated with systemic steroids.
   E Lesions affect the trunk but spare the hands and feet.

Technique

The 'stem' statement should be considered in turn with each item to produce the five complete sentences requiring individual true/false/don't know answers. When answering the question posed by the stem and one item together, all the others items should be disregarded. They should not give any clues to the correct answers and may confuse the issue.

In the example given the answer is true, true, true, true, false but it is important to note that any combination of true and false may occur and there is nothing to prevent all items being true or, equally, all being false.

A total of 300 answers have to be given in the 2 hours allotted and most candidates find that this is the only part of the examination where they finish with plenty of time to spare.

The proportion of the 60 questions devoted to the different areas of general practice knowledge is obviously important as it should influence the time you spend revising each subject. Currently, the breakdown of questions is as shown below:

General medicine	12
Therapeutics	8
Obstetrics and gynaecology	6
Paediatrics	6
Psychiatry	6
Surgical diagnosis	4
ENT	4
Dermatology	4
Eyes	3
Social and legal aspects	3
Epidemiology and statistics	2
Practice organization	2

The question paper itself is in book form but is computer marked by photoelectric scanner. Answers, therefore, have to be recorded on separate computer marking or Opscan sheets (*see* illustration). Each question part has its own true/false lozenge one of which has to be shaded in with the Grade 2B pencil provided. A 'don't know' is indicated by leaving the answer box blank.

4

Please use 2B PENCIL only. Rub out all errors thoroughly.
Mark lozenge like ● <u>Not</u> like this ⌀ ⌀ ⌀

T = True   F = False
Don't know - Leave blank

1	1A T ⊂⊃ F ⊂⊃	1B T ⊂⊃ F ⊂⊃	1C T ⊂⊃ F ⊂⊃	1D T ⊂⊃ F ⊂⊃	1E T ⊂⊃ F ⊂⊃
2	2A T ⊂⊃ F ⊂⊃	2B T ⊂⊃ F ⊂⊃	2C T ⊂⊃ F ⊂⊃	2D T ⊂⊃ F ⊂⊃	2E T ⊂⊃ F ⊂⊃
3	3A T ⊂⊃ F ⊂⊃	3B T ⊂⊃ F ⊂⊃	3C T ⊂⊃ F ⊂⊃	3D T ⊂⊃ F ⊂⊃	3E T ⊂⊃ F ⊂⊃
4	4A T ⊂⊃ F ⊂⊃	4B T ⊂⊃ F ⊂⊃	4C T ⊂⊃ F ⊂⊃	4D T ⊂⊃ F ⊂⊃	4E T ⊂⊃ F ⊂⊃
5	5A T ⊂⊃ F ⊂⊃	5B T ⊂⊃ F ⊂⊃	5C T ⊂⊃ F ⊂⊃	5D T ⊂⊃ F ⊂⊃	5E T ⊂⊃ F ⊂⊃
6	6A T ⊂⊃ F ⊂⊃	6B T ⊂⊃ F ⊂⊃	6C T ⊂⊃ F ⊂⊃	6D T ⊂⊃ F ⊂⊃	6E T ⊂⊃ F ⊂⊃
7	7A T ⊂⊃ F ⊂⊃	7B T ⊂⊃ F ⊂⊃	7C T ⊂⊃ F ⊂⊃	7D T ⊂⊃ F ⊂⊃	7E T ⊂⊃ F ⊂⊃
8	8A T ⊂⊃ F ⊂⊃	8B T ⊂⊃ F ⊂⊃	8C T ⊂⊃ F ⊂⊃	8D T ⊂⊃ F ⊂⊃	8E T ⊂⊃ F ⊂⊃
9	9A T ⊂⊃ F ⊂⊃	9B T ⊂⊃ F ⊂⊃	9C T ⊂⊃ F ⊂⊃	9D T ⊂⊃ F ⊂⊃	9E T ⊂⊃ F ⊂⊃
10	10A T ⊂⊃ F ⊂⊃	10B T ⊂⊃ F ⊂⊃	10C T ⊂⊃ F ⊂⊃	10D T ⊂⊃ F ⊂⊃	10E T ⊂⊃ F ⊂⊃
11	11A T ⊂⊃ F ⊂⊃	11B T ⊂⊃ F ⊂⊃	11C T ⊂⊃ F ⊂⊃	11D T ⊂⊃ F ⊂⊃	11E T ⊂⊃ F ⊂⊃
12	12A T ⊂⊃ F ⊂⊃	12B T ⊂⊃ F ⊂⊃	12C T ⊂⊃ F ⊂⊃	12D T ⊂⊃ F ⊂⊃	12E T ⊂⊃ F ⊂⊃
13	13A T ⊂⊃ F ⊂⊃	13B T ⊂⊃ F ⊂⊃	13C T ⊂⊃ F ⊂⊃	13D T ⊂⊃ F ⊂⊃	13E T ⊂⊃ F ⊂⊃
14	14A T ⊂⊃ F ⊂⊃	14B T ⊂⊃ F ⊂⊃	14C T ⊂⊃ F ⊂⊃	14D T ⊂⊃ F ⊂⊃	14E T ⊂⊃ F ⊂⊃
15	15A T ⊂⊃ F ⊂⊃	15B T ⊂⊃ F ⊂⊃	15C T ⊂⊃ F ⊂⊃	15D T ⊂⊃ F ⊂⊃	15E T ⊂⊃ F ⊂⊃

16	16A T ⊂⊃ F ⊂⊃	16B T ⊂⊃ F ⊂⊃	16C T ⊂⊃ F ⊂⊃	16D T ⊂⊃ F ⊂⊃	16E T ⊂⊃ F ⊂⊃
17	17A T ⊂⊃ F ⊂⊃	17B T ⊂⊃ F ⊂⊃	17C T ⊂⊃ F ⊂⊃	17D T ⊂⊃ F ⊂⊃	17E T ⊂⊃ F ⊂⊃
18	18A T ⊂⊃ F ⊂⊃	18B T ⊂⊃ F ⊂⊃	18C T ⊂⊃ F ⊂⊃	18D T ⊂⊃ F ⊂⊃	18E T ⊂⊃ F ⊂⊃
19	19A T ⊂⊃ F ⊂⊃	19B T ⊂⊃ F ⊂⊃	19C T ⊂⊃ F ⊂⊃	19D T ⊂⊃ F ⊂⊃	19E T ⊂⊃ F ⊂⊃
20	20A T ⊂⊃ F ⊂⊃	20B T ⊂⊃ F ⊂⊃	20C T ⊂⊃ F ⊂⊃	20D T ⊂⊃ F ⊂⊃	20E T ⊂⊃ F ⊂⊃
21	21A T ⊂⊃ F ⊂⊃	21B T ⊂⊃ F ⊂⊃	21C T ⊂⊃ F ⊂⊃	21D T ⊂⊃ F ⊂⊃	21E T ⊂⊃ F ⊂⊃
22	22A T ⊂⊃ F ⊂⊃	22B T ⊂⊃ F ⊂⊃	22C T ⊂⊃ F ⊂⊃	22D T ⊂⊃ F ⊂⊃	22E T ⊂⊃ F ⊂⊃
23	23A T ⊂⊃ F ⊂⊃	23B T ⊂⊃ F ⊂⊃	23C T ⊂⊃ F ⊂⊃	23D T ⊂⊃ F ⊂⊃	23E T ⊂⊃ F ⊂⊃
24	24A T ⊂⊃ F ⊂⊃	24B T ⊂⊃ F ⊂⊃	24C T ⊂⊃ F ⊂⊃	24D T ⊂⊃ F ⊂⊃	24E T ⊂⊃ F ⊂⊃
25	25A T ⊂⊃ F ⊂⊃	25B T ⊂⊃ F ⊂⊃	25C T ⊂⊃ F ⊂⊃	25D T ⊂⊃ F ⊂⊃	25E T ⊂⊃ F ⊂⊃
26	26A T ⊂⊃ F ⊂⊃	26B T ⊂⊃ F ⊂⊃	26C T ⊂⊃ F ⊂⊃	26D T ⊂⊃ F ⊂⊃	26E T ⊂⊃ F ⊂⊃
27	27A T ⊂⊃ F ⊂⊃	27B T ⊂⊃ F ⊂⊃	27C T ⊂⊃ F ⊂⊃	27D T ⊂⊃ F ⊂⊃	27E T ⊂⊃ F ⊂⊃
28	28A T ⊂⊃ F ⊂⊃	28B T ⊂⊃ F ⊂⊃	28C T ⊂⊃ F ⊂⊃	28D T ⊂⊃ F ⊂⊃	28E T ⊂⊃ F ⊂⊃
29	29A T ⊂⊃ F ⊂⊃	29B T ⊂⊃ F ⊂⊃	29C T ⊂⊃ F ⊂⊃	29D T ⊂⊃ F ⊂⊃	29E T ⊂⊃ F ⊂⊃
30	30A T ⊂⊃ F ⊂⊃	30B T ⊂⊃ F ⊂⊃	30C T ⊂⊃ F ⊂⊃	30D T ⊂⊃ F ⊂⊃	30E T ⊂⊃ F ⊂⊃

Marking

The most important point to remember about this paper is that it is marked on a negative marking system. This system is designed to correct for random quessing so that the candidate who knew nothing about the subject and guessed the answers to the questions would on average get half right and half wrong giving a total score of 0.

A correct answer therefore scores +1; an incorrect answer scores −1; and a don't know scores 0. To elaborate, if the totally correct answer to a question were F T T F T, then:

F T T F T	would score	5 out of 5
T T T F T	would score	3 out of 5
D T T F T	would score	4 out of 5
T T T T T	would score	1 out of 5
D T T D T	would score	3 out of 5
T T T T F	would score	−1 out of 5

Random guessing may therefore be penalized with valuable marks lost and your approach to answering should be influenced by this. Of course with many questions you may well have a reasonable idea of the answer, although you are not certain, and in this situation calculated or inspired guessing has been shown to improve candidates' marks.

Wording of questions

So much for the general style of the paper. Now it is worth briefly considering the questions themselves as they can sometimes pose problems. Each part of a question should only be testing one item of knowledge and should use words that are easily understood. Testing of English language knowledge is not an aim and stems and items should be unambiguous. Unfortunately, some questions which appear clear to nearly everyone can appear ambiguous to someone who may have a far more detailed knowledge of an individual field than the question is trying to test or to someone who may just not see what the question is trying to get at. The only advice we can offer in this respect is that there are no trick questions and that they should all be taken at their face

value. If there is genuine doubt in your mind then it is probably safest to mark in a don't know.

In general, words like 'usually', 'often', 'commonly', 'rarely', 'frequently', 'sometimes' are too vague and will not be used (if they are, then they can only be fair if the correct answer is unequivocally false) and too definite words such as 'always' or 'never' will also tend to be avoided as little in medicine is so absolute. Standard terms that have evolved for use in stems, to help overcome the problems of ambiguity, include:

In the majority	Implies in at least 50 per cent of cases
A characteristic feature	One which occurs so often as, usually, to be of some diagnostic significance and, if not present, might lead to doubt being cast on the diagnosis
A recognized feature	Is one that has been reported and that is a fact that a candidate would reasonably be expected to know
A typical feature	Is one that you would expect to be present

Thus all 'characteristic' features are 'recognized' but many 'recognized' features could not be described as 'characteristic'.

If a stem or item does cause confusion and a question does not discriminate between high-scoring and low-scoring candidates then the standard computer analysis of the paper will pick it up and produce an amended score for the question and also allow that question to be replaced in the future. Thus the College's bank of questions is continually being refined to produce even fairer degrees of discrimination between candidates.

Summary of advice

1 Read each question carefully. This may seem obvious but avoidable errors can occur when a question is read quickly and answered without reflection.
2 Remember you are considering the stem and one item together. Disregard the

other items in the question as they have nothing to do with the one you are concentrating on.

3　Answer each item as true or false or leave it blank if you don't know the answer. Make sure your answer is clear and in the correct box.

4　DO NOT RANDOMLY GUESS. Questions you genuinely have no idea about, mark as don't know and move onto more productive areas.

5　Go through the whole filling in the questions of which you are sure then go back to the beginning and spend time thinking out the answers of which you were less confident. Remember, calculated or inspired guessing – when you are fairly certain your answer is correct – is likely to improve your mark.

6　Accept questions at face value. Do not look for hidden catches or tricks. The examiner is not trying to confuse you and the obvious meaning of his statement is the correct one.

7　If you have time to spare at the end check you have put down the answers you meant to and ensure that they are in the correct boxes.

The best way to obtain a good mark is to have as wide a knowledge as possible of the topics being tested in the examination.

However, correct technique in the MCQ will help you not to lose marks unnecessarily.

Further MCQs may be found in the *MCQ Tutor for the MRCGP Examination.* A. J. Moulds and T. L. Bouchier Hayes. London: Heinemann, 1981.

Hints for using the mock tests in this book

Four tests, each of 30 questions, follow. They reflect the subject composition of the College examination and should each be done in 1 hour under examination conditions.

Answers should be filled in on the Opscan sheets provided at each test's start, and self-marking should be strictly based on the negative marking system.

Any answers you strongly disagree with should be checked. We are not infallible but have taken considerable care to be correct!

As in the examination itself, a mark of 50 per cent or more is a pass, 42–50 per cent is borderline and less than 42 per cent worrying. A score of less than 30 per cent either implies you have a tremendous amount of work to do or that you are likely to waste your money sitting the examination.

Please use 2B PENCIL only. Rub out all errors thoroughly.
Mark lozenge like ● <u>Not</u> like this

T = True   F = False
Don't know - Leave blank

	1	A	B	C	D	E
+2	1	1A	1B	1C	1D	1E
+3	2	2A	2B	2C	2D	2E
-2	3	3A	3B	3C	3D	3E
+2	4	4A	4B	4C	4D	4E
+3	5	5A	5B	5C	5D	5E
	6	6A	6B	6C	6D	6E
+3	7	7A	7B	7C	7D	7E
+2	8	8A	8B	8C	8D	8E
+2	9	9A	9B	9C	9D	9E
+1	10	10A	10B	10C	10D	10E
+3	11	11A	11B	11C	11D	11E
+4	12	12A	12B	12C	12D	12E
+1	13	13A	13B	13C	13D	13E
+1	14	14A	14B	14C	14D	14E
+3	15	15A	15B	15C	15D	15E

	16	16A	16B	16C	16D	16E
+4	16	16A	16B	16C	16D	16E
+5	17	17A	17B	17C	17D	17E
0	18	18A	18B	18C	18D	18E
-1	19	19A	19B	19C	19D	19E
0	20	20A	20B	20C	20D	20E
+5	21	21A	21B	21C	21D	21E
+4	22	22A	22B	22C	22D	22E
+1	23	23A	23B	23C	23D	23E
+1	24	24A	24B	24C	24D	24E
+1	25	25A	25B	25C	25D	25E
-1	26	26A	26B	26C	26D	26E
+5	27	27A	27B	27C	27D	27E
+2	28	28A	28B	28C	28D	28E
+3	29	29A	29B	29C	29D	29E
+5	30	30A	30B	30C	30D	30E

62

MCQ
TEST 1

1 In community acquired pneumonia

A The cause is viral in the majority of cases.

B The diagnosis should only be made if there are classic signs of consolidation present.

C A chest X-ray must be obtained as soon as possible.

D The antibiotic of choice is tetracycline.

E Secondary to chickenpox, admission to hospital is likely to be indicated.

2 Recognized antibiotic drug interactions include

A Metronidazole (Flagyl) and alcohol.

B Sulphonamides and phenytoin.

C Tetracyclines and iron preparations.

D Rifampicin and oral contraceptives.

E Cephalosporins and digoxin.

3 Tinnitus

A Commonest cause is wax touching the tympanic membrane.

B Sufferers almost always have some conductive deafness.

C May be effectively treated with tricyclic antidepressants.

D May be treated with a combined hearing aid and sound generating device.

E Will by abolished by section of the acoustic nerves.

4 Phobic anxiety

A May be experienced by the patient at any time or in any place.

B Can be reasoned away.

C Is not seen as irrational by the patient.

D For open spaces is known as claustrophobia.

E Nearly always leads to avoidance of the provoking stimulus.

5 A GP must obtain FPC (Family Practitioner Committee) permission before

A Entering into arrangements with a deputizing service.

B Changing the times he is available for consultation.

C Altering the extent of his practice area.

D Taking on a locum.

E Ceasing to provide maternity services to a woman who still wishes him to look after her.

6 Characteristic features of polymyalgia rheumatica include

A Asymmetrical stiffness.

B Elevated plasma viscosity.

C Good response to oral salicylates.

D Complete recovery within 6–12 months.

E Limb tenderness.

9

7 Miliaria rubra (prickly heat)

A Especially affects the palms and soles.
B Lesions may become pustular.
C If very extensive may lead onto heat stress syndrome.
D Contraindicates the use of topical corticosteroids.
E Can be prevented and treated by cooling.

8 A patient with a corneal abrasion has been fitted with an eyepad

A Complete re-epithelialization is likely to take place within 24 hours.
B The pad should be applied loosely rather than firmly.
C The pad must not be removed for 24 hours for any reason.
D There must be no driving while the pad is in place.
E The pad can be claimed for as a 'dispensed appliance' on the FP34 system.

9 A first episode of genital herpes

A Necessarily implies promiscuity or infidelity.
B In the majority of patients is mild or asymptomatic.
C May be associated with a copious, purulent vaginal discharge.
D Patients should have a towel for their sole use.
E Should be treated with both topical and oral acyclovir (Zovirax).

10 Under the Misuse of Drugs Act and Regulations

A A pharmacist must not dispense a prescription for a controlled drug unless he knows the signature of the prescriber.
B The locked boot of a car would qualify as a safe place of custody for controlled drugs.
C A diagonal line must be drawn across the unused part of any prescription form.
D The police can inspect any GP's register of controlled drugs without notice.
E Suspected addicts must be notified to the Home Office.

11 A patient going to hospital for exercise stress testing could correctly be advised that the test

A Will take place on a bicycle ergometer.
B Can only be carried out if he or she is fit.
C Is totally without risk.
D Can be stopped at any stage.
E Is not painful, in itself, in any way.

12 In the treatment of infertility, clomiphene citrate (Clomid)

A Could be used in a woman with polycystic ovary syndrome.
B Dosage regimen is 50 mg daily for 5 days.
C Recognized side effects include visual disturbance.
D Will improve the ovulation rate by about 80 per cent.
E If successful is associated with an increased multiple pregnancy rate.

13 Chondromalacia patellae

A Pain is aggravated by prolonged sitting with knees flexed beyond 90 degrees.
B Diagnosis should not be made in the absence of patellofemoral crepitus.
C Is a recognized cause of episodes of momentary locking of the knee.
D Diagnosis should be confirmed by arthroscopy.
E Symptoms may be relieved by intensive vastus medialis muscle exercises.

14 Non-accidental injury in children

A Is commoner in children from social classes 4 and 5.
B Should be strongly suspected in any school-age child with more than two bruises.
C In the majority of cases involves face or head injury.
D Includes retinal haemorrhage from severe shaking.
E If only suspected by the GP is best managed by practice observation.

15 The risk of developing breast cancer is increased in women who

A Have had four or more children.
B Had a late menarche or early menopause.

C Have ever taken the combined contraceptive pill.

D Have a past history of benign breast disease which required biopsy.

E Have a family history of breast cancer.

16 Asymptomatic microscopic haematuria found on urine stick testing

A Should be ignored if urine microscopy fails to confirm the presence of red cells.

B In a young patient, may be due to athletic activities.

C In patients over 40, full urological investigation is mandatory.

D In a patient on anticoagulants, can safely be ignored.

E If investigated in patients under 40, only 2 per cent will prove to have a serious urological lesion.

17 Tinea capitis

A Causes red, scaling, inflamed patches in the scalp.

B Affects children rather than adults.

C Cannot spread from person to person.

D Hair loss is always temporary.

E Treatment of choice is griseofulvin.

18 Features which would support a diagnosis of school phobia rather than of truancy include

A Child not emotionally distressed.

B High standard of school work when at school.

C Parents of social class 1 and 2.

D Child stays away from home as well as from school.

E A history of antisocial behaviour in the family.

19 Nausea and vomiting in pregnancy

A Reach their peak at about 8 weeks' gestation.

B Affects about one in three pregnant women.

C Is as likely to occur in the evening as in the morning.

D In some patients can be helped by eating a biscuit before rising in the morning.

E Antiemetic of choice is pyridoxine.

20 When using centile charts to assess whether a child is growing normally or not, remember

A Normal children grow in height along lines parallel to the centiles.

B Children whose heights are above the 97th centile or below the 3rd are abnormal.

C A child on the 90th height centile should also be on the 90th weight centile.

D Serial height measurements should normally be taken 6 months apart.

E The 50th centile is the mean.

21 Epilepsy

A Each year in the UK, 20 000 new cases present.

B Diagnosis can only be made if the EEG is abnormal.

C Of focal onset requires further investigation.

D Drugs should be given at intervals of approximately their half-life.

E Patients should be advised not to sit too close to a TV set.

22 Digoxin therapy

A In atrial fibrillation, apical rate should always be used as clinical measure of response.

B Absolute contraindications include impaired renal function.

C In cardiac failure, tolerance to treatment develops.

D Toxicity should only be diagnosed where serum levels are high.

E Toxic effects of nausea and vomiting should improve within 24 hours of withdrawing the drug or reducing the dose.

23 Maldescended testes

A Are more likely if the scrotal skin is less rugose on one side.

B If examination is inconclusive, asking the child to squat for re-examination may be helpful.

C If retractile, require no treatment.

D Undescended in men after puberty are best treated with surgical exploration and orchidectomy.

E If undescended, should be fixed in the scrotum between 5 and 7 years of age.

24 Measles vaccine

A May be used up to 48 hours after being reconstituted.

B May prevent measles if given up to 5 days after exposure.

C Use is recommended for children who have had convulsions.

D Use would be contraindicated in a child intermittently using 1% hydrocortisone cream for eczema.

E Seroconversion occurs in 95 per cent of recipients.

25 For emergency compulsory hospital admission under Section 4 of the Mental Health Act, the patient

A Must have been seen within 24 hours by the applicants.

B Can be detained for a maximum of 28 days.

C Has the right of appeal to a review tribunal.

D Must be admitted to hospital within 24 hours of sectioning.

E Applicant can be approved social worker or any relative.

26 Hyperosmolar non-ketotic hyperglycaemic diabetic patients

A Are far more likely to be insulin dependent than not.

B Hyperventilate.

C Have little or no ketonuria.

D Normally present with a history of confused behaviour leading to coma.

E Tend to be insulin resistant.

27 In the treatment of head lice, malathion products (Derbac-M, Prioderm, Suleo-M)

A Lotion should remain on the head for 10–15 minutes only.

B Should be used daily for at least 7 days.

C May have a residual action which prevents early reinfection.

D Should be used in preference to gamma benzene hexachloride products.

E After use, patients should be advised not to use hair brushes.

28 Submandibular gland or duct calculi

A Pain characteristically subsides shortly after eating.

B Are easily palpable.

C May present with swelling in the upper part of the anterior triangle of the neck.

D In the majority of cases are radiolucent.

E May be able to be removed intraorally.

29 Premature ejaculators

A Are defined as men who cannot 'last' more than 10 minutes during coitus.

B Characteristically ejaculate quickly in association with poor erection.

C In some cases may be helped by correction of poor sex technique.

D In some cases may be helped by squeeze technique or Seman's manoeuvre.

E May be helped by clomipramine (Anafranil) 10 mg at 6 p.m.

30 After delivery

A Natural infertility will last for as long as any breast feeding is taking place.

B IUDs must not be inserted for at least 3 months.

C Diaphragms used prior to pregnancy should not be used before 6 weeks.

D Postpartum sterilization is best carried out within 1–2 days.

E The Pill should not be started until the first period.

THE ANSWERS TO MCQ TEST 1 BEGIN ON PAGE 31

14

Please use 2B PENCIL only. Rub out all errors thoroughly.
Mark lozenge like ● Not like this ⊘ ⊘ ⊗

T = True   F = False
Don't know - Leave blank

1	1A T◯ F◯	1B T◯ F◯	1C T◯ F◯	1D T◯ F◯	1E T◯ F◯
2	2A T◯ F◯	2B T◯ F◯	2C T◯ F◯	2D T◯ F◯	2E T◯ F◯
3	3A T◯ F◯	3B T◯ F◯	3C T◯ F◯	3D T◯ F◯	3E T◯ F◯
4	4A T◯ F◯	4B T◯ F◯	4C T◯ F◯	4D T◯ F◯	4E T◯ F◯
5	5A T◯ F◯	5B T◯ F◯	5C T◯ F◯	5D T◯ F◯	5E T◯ F◯
6	6A T◯ F◯	6B T◯ F◯	6C T◯ F◯	6D T◯ F◯	6E T◯ F◯
7	7A T◯ F◯	7B T◯ F◯	7C T◯ F◯	7D T◯ F◯	7E T◯ F◯
8	8A T◯ F◯	8B T◯ F◯	8C T◯ F◯	8D T◯ F◯	8E T◯ F◯
9	9A T◯ F◯	9B T◯ F◯	9C T◯ F◯	9D T◯ F◯	9E T◯ F◯
10	10A T◯ F◯	10B T◯ F◯	10C T◯ F◯	10D T◯ F◯	10E T◯ F◯
11	11A T◯ F◯	11B T◯ F◯	11C T◯ F◯	11D T◯ F◯	11E T◯ F◯
12	12A T◯ F◯	12B T◯ F◯	12C T◯ F◯	12D T◯ F◯	12E T◯ F◯
13	13A T◯ F◯	13B T◯ F◯	13C T◯ F◯	13D T◯ F◯	13E T◯ F◯
14	14A T◯ F◯	14B T◯ F◯	14C T◯ F◯	14D T◯ F◯	14E T◯ F◯
15	15A T◯ F◯	15B T◯ F◯	15C T◯ F◯	15D T◯ F◯	15E T◯ F◯
16	16A T◯ F◯	16B T◯ F◯	16C T◯ F◯	16D T◯ F◯	16E T◯ F◯
17	17A T◯ F◯	17B T◯ F◯	17C T◯ F◯	17D T◯ F◯	17E T◯ F◯
18	18A T◯ F◯	18B T◯ F◯	18C T◯ F◯	18D T◯ F◯	18E T◯ F◯
19	19A T◯ F◯	19B T◯ F◯	19C T◯ F◯	19D T◯ F◯	19E T◯ F◯
20	20A T◯ F◯	20B T◯ F◯	20C T◯ F◯	20D T◯ F◯	20E T◯ F◯
21	21A T◯ F◯	21B T◯ F◯	21C T◯ F◯	21D T◯ F◯	21E T◯ F◯
22	22A T◯ F◯	22B T◯ F◯	22C T◯ F◯	22D T◯ F◯	22E T◯ F◯
23	23A T◯ F◯	23B T◯ F◯	23C T◯ F◯	23D T◯ F◯	23E T◯ F◯
24	24A T◯ F◯	24B T◯ F◯	24C T◯ F◯	24D T◯ F◯	24E T◯ F◯
25	25A T◯ F◯	25B T◯ F◯	25C T◯ F◯	25D T◯ F◯	25E T◯ F◯
26	26A T◯ F◯	26B T◯ F◯	26C T◯ F◯	26D T◯ F◯	26E T◯ F◯
27	27A T◯ F◯	27B T◯ F◯	27C T◯ F◯	27D T◯ F◯	27E T◯ F◯
28	28A T◯ F◯	28B T◯ F◯	28C T◯ F◯	28D T◯ F◯	28E T◯ F◯
29	29A T◯ F◯	29B T◯ F◯	29C T◯ F◯	29D T◯ F◯	29E T◯ F◯
30	30A T◯ F◯	30B T◯ F◯	30C T◯ F◯	30D T◯ F◯	30E T◯ F◯

MCQ
TEST 2

Time allowed – one hour

All questions must be answered by filling in the true/false or don't know boxes on the computer marking sheet

1 *Ulcerative colitis patients*

A Are invariably smokers.
B With proctitis alone may present with constipation.
C With mild to moderate symptoms, may have no abnormality to find on surgery examination.
D Relapse rate is markedly decreased by sulphasalazine 1 g twice daily, taken long term.
E Should undergo regular screening by barium enema (because of risk of developing cancer).

2 *In an elderly patient in heart failure being treated with a thiazide diuretic, the following side effects may occur*

A Hypoglycaemia.
B Hypernatraemia.
C Incontinence.
D Gout.
E Increased urinary calcium excretion.

3 *Dental abscesses*

A Associated tooth may be tender on palpation.
B May cause trismus.
C In most cases will not respond to penicillin.
D Should not be incised unless the patient has been on antibiotics for at least 48 hours.

E Treated by a GP attract the emergency dental item of service payment.

4 *With normal/average development, an 18-month-old child should be able to*

A Spontaneously join two or three words together to make a sentence.
B Cast objects, one after another.
C Turn the pages of a book two or three at a time.
D Be mainly dry by day.
E Run.

5 *In a 16-year-old girl with primary dysmenorrhoea*

A Periods will have been painful since the menarche.
B The pain will start several days before the flow.
C Pelvic examination is mandatory.
D Aspirin is unlikely to be helpful.
E The treatment of choice is dilatation of the cervix.

6 *Recognized features of senile (idiopathic) osteoporosis include*

A Back pain worsened by flexing the spine.
B Pseudofractures.
C Markedly elevated serum alkaline phosphatase levels.
D Loss of sitting height.

E A transverse skin crease across the upper abdomen above the umbilicus.

7 In the prophylaxis of migraine, pizotifen (Sanomigran)

A Use may cause increase in weight.
B Patients should be warned that the drug may impair their ability to drive.
C Normal adult dose of 1.5 mg may be taken in one dose at night.
D If effective, may be continued for years.
E Works because it is an ergot derivative.

8 Successful community care for chronic schizophrenics is likely to involve

A Maintenance administration of neuroleptic medication.
B As much stimulation and change as possible to retrain the patient for work.
C Visits from the community psychiatric nurse.
D Reassurance and support for relatives.
E Seeing the GP every 2 months or so.

9 Supraspinatus tendinitis

A Most commonly affects younger sportsmen.
B Typically presents with a complaint of painful initiation of abduction.
C Mainstay of treatment is to rest the shoulder for 2–3 weeks.
D May be helped by steroid injected into the subacromial bursa.
E If not helped by medical management may be effectively treated surgically.

10 A social security doctor's special statement (form Med 5)

A Must not be for more than 1 month.
B May be issued by one partner for a patient seen by another partner.
C May be issued on the basis of a hospital doctor's report which is not more than 3 months old.
D Should have the doctor's name and address stamped on it.
E Must always state the precise diagnosis.

11 Haemophiliacs

A Who have teeth removed bleed abnormally in the dentist's chair.
B Can be diagnosed prenatally at 16–20 weeks' gestation.
C Cannot be the sons of haemophiliac men.
D Haemarthroses will resolve with injections of clotting factor concentrates.
E With AIDS antibodies should be treated as contagious and be advised to eat alone and have no physical contact with other people.

12 Fifth disease (erythema infectiosum)

A Peak attack rates are in the 4–10 year age group.
B Facial rash makes the cheeks hyperaemic and swollen.
C Causes no prodromal symptoms.
D Rash characteristically lasts for up to 1 week.
E Affected child must be kept off school until the rash has cleared.

13 Characteristic features of endogenous depression include

A Abrupt onset.
B Sad facial expression.
C Looseness of the bowels.
D Disturbed sleep.
E Weight gain.

14 Fissure in ano

A Fissure is typically situated in the anterior midline.
B Pain is only present at or for a short time after defaecation.
C Is a recognized cause of rectal bleeding.
D Contraindicates the use of local anaesthetic ointments.
E May be effectively treated by anal stretch.

15 Community Health Councils

A Were first established in 1948 when the NHS was set up.
B Are non-statutory bodies.
C Are funded by the FPCs in their area.
D Members are elected.
E Provide members of the public with a channel for complaints against the health service.

16 Multiple sclerosis

A Even clinically silent lesions can be identified on CT scan.

B Leads rapidly and inevitably to a wheelchair existence.

C Sufferers should be strongly advised not to get pregnant.

D Associated depression may be effectively treated with amitriptyline in a single bedtime dose.

E Frequency of relapses is lessened by long-term oral corticosteroid therapy.

17 In breast cancer, tamoxifen

A Elimination half-life is about 2 weeks.

B In most postmenopausal women causes no unwanted effects.

C Therapy may cause hypercalcaemia.

D Use is contraindicated when carcinoma is recurrent.

E Used as an adjuvant after adequate local therapy may prolong survival.

18 Characteristic features of chronic suppurative otitis media include

A Vertigo.

B Earache.

C Deafness.

D Cholesteatoma.

E Recurrent episodes of foul smelling discharge.

19 In croup

A In contrast to epiglottitis, cough and stridor are loud.

B Respiratory rate correlates with degree of hypoxia.

C Amoxycillin is the antibiotic of choice.

D Highest incidence is found among 4–7 year olds.

E A cold, misty environment will help.

20 Requirements of a good repeat prescribing system include

A Not routinely used for psychotropic drugs.

B Patients able to get drugs within 24 hours of a request.

C All prescriptions written out by receptionists for doctor's signature.

D A recall system which is clear to both patients and staff.

E A therapy card held in the patient's notes.

21 Mesothelioma

A Lag between exposure to asbestos and disease is normally 10–15 years.

B Only rarely causes chest pain.

C Characteristically causes finger clubbing.

D Median survival from onset of symptoms is about 1 year whatever treatment is given.

E May give rise to progressive dyspnoea.

22 Rhinophyma

A Is as common in females as males.

B Characteristically causes nasal obstruction.

C Condition does not fluctuate with vascular dilatation.

D Is most effectively treated with oral antibiotics such as oxytetracycline.

E May be treated with repeated application of liquid nitrogen or solid carbon dioxide.

23 Indecent exposers who commit exhibitionismus rigidus

A Are dirty men in raincoats.

B In most cases are married.

C Gain pleasure from the act.

D Are more likely to indulge in other sexual offences than flaccid exhibitionists.

E If convicted can be fined up to £400.

24 The progestogen-only Pill

A Acts to make the endometrium unreceptive to the implantation of the fertilized ovum.

B Failure rate increases with duration of use.

C Should be taken regularly about 1 hour before intercourse usually takes place.

D Should not be prescribed to a woman who wears contact lenses.

E Should be stopped 4–6 weeks before major surgery.

25 It is correct to say that

A The prevalence of high blood pressure, diagnosed on the basis of sphygmomanometric readings, is over 20 per cent in adults over 30 years old.

B Fifty per cent of all hypertensives in the community are undiagnosed.

C Over 80 per cent of all newly diagnosed hypertensives are under 60 years old when first diagnosed.

D In hypertensives first diagnosed over the age of 60 years, the expected mortality rates are scarcely above those expected in a normal population.

E The major risk in hypertensives is death from ischaemic heart disease.

26 The erythrocyte sedimentation rate

A Normal limit in men is age in years divided by two.

B Is lowered in patients taking NSAIDs.

C May be moderately elevated if the serum cholesterol is elevated.

D For accuracy should always be performed in the laboratory.

E If over 100 mm/h for 1 month or more, is associated with a poor prognosis.

27 Non-immune travellers going to stay in a malarious area should be advised that antimalarial drugs

A Do not need to be taken by babies.

B Should be taken for at least 1 week prior to exposure.

C Taken regularly will be 100 per cent effective.

D Should be taken for at least 4 weeks after leaving the malarious areas.

E Are not available on NHS prescription.

28 Characteristic features of ectopic pregnancy include

A Unilateral pelvic pain.

B Brown vaginal discharge.

C Negative pregnancy test.

D Pyrexia.

E Referred pain at the shoulder tips.

29 In a baby with sticky eyes from congenital non-patency of the lacrimal drainage apparatus

A Watering of the eye may begin within a few days of birth.

B Pressure on the lacrimal sac may cause mucus to be expressed into the eye.

C Swabs should always be taken before using antibiotic ointments.

D Non-treatment might lead to future visual impairment.

E Spontaneous resolution after about 9 months is the rule.

30 Children with coeliac disease

A Normally present before they are 2 years old.

B May become constipated.

C Although losing weight remain cheerful and active.

D Gluten-free diet excludes all foods containing wheat, rye and barley.

E On treatment, height and weight return to normal centiles within 3 months or so.

THE ANSWERS TO MCQ TEST 2 BEGIN ON PAGE 34

Please use 2B PENCIL only. Rub out all errors thoroughly.
Mark lozenge like ● Not like this ⊘ ⊘ ⊗

T = True   F = False
Don't know - Leave blank

1	1A	1B	1C	1D	1E
	T ⊂⊃	T ⊂⊃	T ⊂⊃	T ⊂⊃	T ⊂⊃
	F ⊂⊃	F ⊂⊃	F ⊂⊃	F ⊂⊃	F ⊂⊃
2	2A	2B	2C	2D	2E
	T ⊂⊃	T ⊂⊃	T ⊂⊃	T ⊂⊃	T ⊂⊃
	F ⊂⊃	F ⊂⊃	F ⊂⊃	F ⊂⊃	F ⊂⊃
3	3A	3B	3C	3D	3E
	T ⊂⊃	T ⊂⊃	T ⊂⊃	T ⊂⊃	T ⊂⊃
	F ⊂⊃	F ⊂⊃	F ⊂⊃	F ⊂⊃	F ⊂⊃
4	4A	4B	4C	4D	4E
	T ⊂⊃	T ⊂⊃	T ⊂⊃	T ⊂⊃	T ⊂⊃
	F ⊂⊃	F ⊂⊃	F ⊂⊃	F ⊂⊃	F ⊂⊃
5	5A	5B	5C	5D	5E
	T ⊂⊃	T ⊂⊃	T ⊂⊃	T ⊂⊃	T ⊂⊃
	F ⊂⊃	F ⊂⊃	F ⊂⊃	F ⊂⊃	F ⊂⊃
6	6A	6B	6C	6D	6E
	T ⊂⊃	T ⊂⊃	T ⊂⊃	T ⊂⊃	T ⊂⊃
	F ⊂⊃	F ⊂⊃	F ⊂⊃	F ⊂⊃	F ⊂⊃
7	7A	7B	7C	7D	7E
	T ⊂⊃	T ⊂⊃	T ⊂⊃	T ⊂⊃	T ⊂⊃
	F ⊂⊃	F ⊂⊃	F ⊂⊃	F ⊂⊃	F ⊂⊃
8	8A	8B	8C	8D	8E
	T ⊂⊃	T ⊂⊃	T ⊂⊃	T ⊂⊃	T ⊂⊃
	F ⊂⊃	F ⊂⊃	F ⊂⊃	F ⊂⊃	F ⊂⊃
9	9A	9B	9C	9D	9E
	T ⊂⊃	T ⊂⊃	T ⊂⊃	T ⊂⊃	T ⊂⊃
	F ⊂⊃	F ⊂⊃	F ⊂⊃	F ⊂⊃	F ⊂⊃
10	10A	10B	10C	10D	10E
	T ⊂⊃	T ⊂⊃	T ⊂⊃	T ⊂⊃	T ⊂⊃
	F ⊂⊃	F ⊂⊃	F ⊂⊃	F ⊂⊃	F ⊂⊃
11	11A	11B	11C	11D	11E
	T ⊂⊃	T ⊂⊃	T ⊂⊃	T ⊂⊃	T ⊂⊃
	F ⊂⊃	F ⊂⊃	F ⊂⊃	F ⊂⊃	F ⊂⊃
12	12A	12B	12C	12D	12E
	T ⊂⊃	T ⊂⊃	T ⊂⊃	T ⊂⊃	T ⊂⊃
	F ⊂⊃	F ⊂⊃	F ⊂⊃	F ⊂⊃	F ⊂⊃
13	13A	13B	13C	13D	13E
	T ⊂⊃	T ⊂⊃	T ⊂⊃	T ⊂⊃	T ⊂⊃
	F ⊂⊃	F ⊂⊃	F ⊂⊃	F ⊂⊃	F ⊂⊃
14	14A	14B	14C	14D	14E
	T ⊂⊃	T ⊂⊃	T ⊂⊃	T ⊂⊃	T ⊂⊃
	F ⊂⊃	F ⊂⊃	F ⊂⊃	F ⊂⊃	F ⊂⊃
15	15A	15B	15C	15D	15E
	T ⊂⊃	T ⊂⊃	T ⊂⊃	T ⊂⊃	T ⊂⊃
	F ⊂⊃	F ⊂⊃	F ⊂⊃	F ⊂⊃	F ⊂⊃

16	16A	16B	16C	16D	16E
	T ⊂⊃	T ⊂⊃	T ⊂⊃	T ⊂⊃	T ⊂⊃
	F ⊂⊃	F ⊂⊃	F ⊂⊃	F ⊂⊃	F ⊂⊃
17	17A	17B	17C	17D	17E
	T ⊂⊃	T ⊂⊃	T ⊂⊃	T ⊂⊃	T ⊂⊃
	F ⊂⊃	F ⊂⊃	F ⊂⊃	F ⊂⊃	F ⊂⊃
18	18A	18B	18C	18D	18E
	T ⊂⊃	T ⊂⊃	T ⊂⊃	T ⊂⊃	T ⊂⊃
	F ⊂⊃	F ⊂⊃	F ⊂⊃	F ⊂⊃	F ⊂⊃
19	19A	19B	19C	19D	19E
	T ⊂⊃	T ⊂⊃	T ⊂⊃	T ⊂⊃	T ⊂⊃
	F ⊂⊃	F ⊂⊃	F ⊂⊃	F ⊂⊃	F ⊂⊃
20	20A	20B	20C	20D	20E
	T ⊂⊃	T ⊂⊃	T ⊂⊃	T ⊂⊃	T ⊂⊃
	F ⊂⊃	F ⊂⊃	F ⊂⊃	F ⊂⊃	F ⊂⊃
21	21A	21B	21C	21D	21E
	T ⊂⊃	T ⊂⊃	T ⊂⊃	T ⊂⊃	T ⊂⊃
	F ⊂⊃	F ⊂⊃	F ⊂⊃	F ⊂⊃	F ⊂⊃
22	22A	22B	22C	22D	22E
	T ⊂⊃	T ⊂⊃	T ⊂⊃	T ⊂⊃	T ⊂⊃
	F ⊂⊃	F ⊂⊃	F ⊂⊃	F ⊂⊃	F ⊂⊃
23	23A	23B	23C	23D	23E
	T ⊂⊃	T ⊂⊃	T ⊂⊃	T ⊂⊃	T ⊂⊃
	F ⊂⊃	F ⊂⊃	F ⊂⊃	F ⊂⊃	F ⊂⊃
24	24A	24B	24C	24D	24E
	T ⊂⊃	T ⊂⊃	T ⊂⊃	T ⊂⊃	T ⊂⊃
	F ⊂⊃	F ⊂⊃	F ⊂⊃	F ⊂⊃	F ⊂⊃
25	25A	25B	25C	25D	25E
	T ⊂⊃	T ⊂⊃	T ⊂⊃	T ⊂⊃	T ⊂⊃
	F ⊂⊃	F ⊂⊃	F ⊂⊃	F ⊂⊃	F ⊂⊃
26	26A	26B	26C	26D	26E
	T ⊂⊃	T ⊂⊃	T ⊂⊃	T ⊂⊃	T ⊂⊃
	F ⊂⊃	F ⊂⊃	F ⊂⊃	F ⊂⊃	F ⊂⊃
27	27A	27B	27C	27D	27E
	T ⊂⊃	T ⊂⊃	T ⊂⊃	T ⊂⊃	T ⊂⊃
	F ⊂⊃	F ⊂⊃	F ⊂⊃	F ⊂⊃	F ⊂⊃
28	28A	28B	28C	28D	28E
	T ⊂⊃	T ⊂⊃	T ⊂⊃	T ⊂⊃	T ⊂⊃
	F ⊂⊃	F ⊂⊃	F ⊂⊃	F ⊂⊃	F ⊂⊃
29	29A	29B	29C	29D	29E
	T ⊂⊃	T ⊂⊃	T ⊂⊃	T ⊂⊃	T ⊂⊃
	F ⊂⊃	F ⊂⊃	F ⊂⊃	F ⊂⊃	F ⊂⊃
30	30A	30B	30C	30D	30E
	T ⊂⊃	T ⊂⊃	T ⊂⊃	T ⊂⊃	T ⊂⊃
	F ⊂⊃	F ⊂⊃	F ⊂⊃	F ⊂⊃	F ⊂⊃

MCQ
TEST 3

Time allowed – one hour

All questions must be answered by filling in the true/false or don't know boxes on the computer marking sheet

1 Reiter's syndrome

A Affects men but not women.
B Infecting organism causing the urethritis does not differ from that causing uncomplicated non-gonococcal urethritis.
C Arthritis is seropositive.
D Urethritis is followed in about one in three cases by iritis.
E Recognized complications include circinate balanitis.

2 Recognized side effects of nifedipine (Adalat) therapy include

A Ankle swelling.
B Dizziness.
C Precipitation of gout.
D Precipitation of angina.
E Cramps.

3 Glue ear

A Affects 10 per cent of all children at some time in their early years.
B Loss of hearing may fluctuate with colds.
C Level of deafness is normally about 60–70 decibels.
D Tympanic membrane is typically dull.
E Leads to permanent deafness in one in 500 cases.

4 After haemorrhoidectomy

A Patients will be kept in hospital for 7–10 days.
B Bulk laxatives are contraindicated.
C Secondary haemorrhage is most likely at 7–10 days.
D Pain is characteristically significantly worse than after an operation such as appendicectomy.
E Pain may be less in the patient with a comparatively lax anal spincter.

5 The combined Pill must be discontinued in a woman who develops

A Headaches in the Pill withdrawal interval.
B Migraine with transient episodes of weakness.
C Infective hepatitis.
D Gastroenteritis.
E Varicose veins.

6 Characteristic features of heartburn include

A Retrosternal discomfort.
B Radiation down the arms.
C Better after meals.
D Worsened by cold drinks.
E Food sticking.

21

7 In the treatment of delerium in the elderly, thioridazine (Melleril)

A Is more effective if given after the delerium has become intense rather than prophylactically.
B Rarely, may produce an increase in confusion.
C Use is contraindicated in patients with Parkinson's disease.
D Initial dose would be 100–200 mg/day.
E Use does not obviate the need for as reassuring an environment for the patient as possible.

8 Arc eye (welder's flash)

A Is due to exposure to infrared light.
B Follows within 1–2 hours of unguarded exposure to a welding arc.
C Does not cause photophobia.
D Fluorescein staining will show the cornea stippled with punctate erosions.
E Contraindicates the use of 1% amethocaine drops.

9 'Growing pains' in childhood

A Peak incidence is between 6 and 13 years.
B May affect legs, arms or trunk.
C In most cases occur during the night.
D Examination, when in pain, reveals tender muscles.
E Management consists of instructing the parent to rub the affected part.

10 Characteristic features of tennis elbow include

A Parasthesiae in the arm.
B Pain radiating down posterolateral aspect of forearm.
C Pain on resisted extension of the wrist.
D Periosteal reaction at the epicondyle visible on X-ray.
E Relief, after a few hours, of symptoms with local steroid injection.

11 In acute pancreatitis

A Alcohol excess is the cause in most cases.
B Serum amylase levels are directly proportional to the severity of the disease.
C Abdominal examination is characteristically negative.
D Pain will be relieved by antacids.
E Urgent laparotomy is the treatment of choice.

12 In a patient taking warfarin

A Risk of haemorrhage is directly proportional to degree of anticoagulant control.
B Dihydrocodeine can be safely prescribed.
C Metronidazole (Flagyl) will inhibit warfarin metabolism.
D Ranitidine (Zantac) would be the drug of choice for an associated peptic ulcer.
E If oral contraception were essential then the progestogen-only Pill would be better than the Pill itself.

13 Postnatal depression

A May occur at any time in the first postpartum year.
B May present with frequent visits for minor physical complaints.
C Is most likely to occur in primips.
D Does not respond to antidepressant drugs.
E Is characteristically associated with hallucinations.

14 A patient should be advised not to apply for or to hold a public service vehicle licence if he or she has

A Defective colour vision.
B Hypertension effectively controlled by beta-blockers.
C Insulin-dependent diabetes.
D Not been free from any epileptic attack since reaching the age of 3 years.
E Parkinson's disease.

15 Carcinoma of the vulva

A May arise at the site of pre-existing leukoplakia.
B Peak incidence is in 40–60 year olds.
C Characteristically presents with pain.
D Treatment of choice is radiotherapy.
E Does not metastasize.

16 Rubella HI (haemagglutination inhibition) antibodies

A In the majority of cases will be detectable within a week of the onset of the rash.

B Are less reliable diagnostically than isolation of the virus.

C Detectable at low titre (<100 units) within 1 week of a rubella-like illness is diagnostic of rubella.

D Detectable in serum taken within 10 days of contact with a rubella-like illness represent residual antibodies from a past infection.

E Are routinely measured to test that immunization has 'taken'.

17 Chilblains (erythema pernio)

A Are primarily a condition of old age.

B Do not itch.

C May develop on thighs and buttocks.

D Are white in colour.

E Sufferers should be advised to apply local heat to the chilblain area, as soon as they get in from the cold.

18 Autistic children

A Are, in the majority of cases, of normal intelligence.

B Cannot be cured.

C Have problems in understanding and using any form of communication.

D Characteristically sleep well.

E Are suffering from a specific disease with a single aetiology.

19 Pre-eclamptic toxaemia (PET) characteristically

A Affects multips rather than primips.

B Develops in the last few weeks of pregnancy.

C Progresses rapidly to eclampsia.

D Is more likely to occur in diabetics.

E Presents with headaches and visual disturbance.

20 Attendance allowance may be paid

A For patients who need frequent attendance to prevent damage to themselves or others.

B Only when the need has existed for 6 months.

C For patients living in a local authority home.

D At a higher rate if attention is needed by night as well as by day.

E Only up to an upper age limit of 75 years.

21 In a patient with an indwelling catheter for long-term bladder drainage, for best results

A Regular routine urine cultures should be taken.

B Use the largest (comfortable) catheter size possible.

C Empty the drainage bag as infrequently as possible.

D Use no more than 10 ml of water in the balloon.

E Change the catheter routinely every 6–8 weeks.

22 Drug placebo effects

A Are felt immediately.

B Can only benefit the patient.

C Are greater in children than in adults.

D Are enhanced by the conviction and confidence with which the doctor prescribes.

E May be tested in double-blind controlled trials.

23 Characteristic features of Menière's disease include

A Positive family history.

B Progressive decline in hearing.

C Tinnitus decreases during episodes of vertigo.

D Starts unilaterally.

E Loss of consciousness during attacks.

24 In child sexual abuse

A Up to 50 per cent of perpetrators are well known to the child.

B The GP must protect the confidentiality of an adult patient who is also a child abuser.

C Uncorroborated allegations by children should not be believed.

D Medical examination should be carried out by a forensically experienced practitioner.

E Cases are best managed within a multidisciplinary team.

25 Under the Employment Protection Act 1975, a receptionist

A Even if she is the GP's spouse must be given a written contract.

B Is entitled to take part in Trade Union activities within working hours.

C Has the right to take paid time off work for antenatal care.

D Must be given a minimum of 20 days' paid holiday a year.

E Must be given an itemized pay statement.

26 In diabetics, glycosylated haemoglobin (HbA1)

A Gives information regarding control for past 8–12 months.

B Values of more than 10 per cent are unacceptable and show need for radical change in management.

C Should be estimated on a fasting blood sample.

D Value may be lowered if there is a shortened red cell survival time.

E Levels if normal can only mean that control is good.

27 In scabies

A Maximum discomfort is usually experienced just after retiring for the night.

B Holding hands is the normal method of transfer of infection.

C Disease is never spread by fomites.

D For treatment, gamma benzene hexachloride (Esoderm, Lorexane, Quellada) should be preferred to benzyl benzoate (Ascabiol).

E Advice to take a hot bath before treatment is soundly based.

28 Factors suggesting that a patient who attempted suicide had genuine suicidal intent include

A Telling others about intention before the attempt.

B Event timed so that intervention unlikely.

C Preparations made in anticipation of death.

D Alcohol used as part of the attempt.

E Leaving a suicide note.

29 An infant should not be given its first triple and polio if there is a history of

A Prematurity and low birth weight.

B Respiratory distress syndrome.

C Congenital heart defect.

D Never free from snuffles.

E A cousin with fits.

30 It is correct to say that

A A standard unit of alcohol is defined as 1 pint of beer or 2 glasses of sherry.

B GPs have a mortality rate from cirrhosis less than the national average.

C Two in three excessive drinkers will have an increased red cell MCV.

D Fifty per cent of drivers killed in road traffic accidents are intoxicated.

E Each GP has about 100 alcoholics on his or her list.

THE ANSWERS TO MCQ TEST 3 BEGIN ON PAGE 38

26

Please use 2B PENCIL only. Rub out all errors thoroughly.
Mark lozenge like ● Not like this ⊘ ⊘ ⊗

T = True   F = False
Don't know · Leave blank

1	1A T◯ F◯	1B T◯ F◯	1C T◯ F◯	1D T◯ F◯	1E T◯ F◯
2	2A T◯ F◯	2B T◯ F◯	2C T◯ F◯	2D T◯ F◯	2E T◯ F◯
3	3A T◯ F◯	3B T◯ F◯	3C T◯ F◯	3D T◯ F◯	3E T◯ F◯
4	4A T◯ F◯	4B T◯ F◯	4C T◯ F◯	4D T◯ F◯	4E T◯ F◯
5	5A T◯ F◯	5B T◯ F◯	5C T◯ F◯	5D T◯ F◯	5E T◯ F◯
6	6A T◯ F◯	6B T◯ F◯	6C T◯ F◯	6D T◯ F◯	6E T◯ F◯
7	7A T◯ F◯	7B T◯ F◯	7C T◯ F◯	7D T◯ F◯	7E T◯ F◯
8	8A T◯ F◯	8B T◯ F◯	8C T◯ F◯	8D T◯ F◯	8E T◯ F◯
9	9A T◯ F◯	9B T◯ F◯	9C T◯ F◯	9D T◯ F◯	9E T◯ F◯
10	10A T◯ F◯	10B T◯ F◯	10C T◯ F◯	10D T◯ F◯	10E T◯ F◯
11	11A T◯ F◯	11B T◯ F◯	11C T◯ F◯	11D T◯ F◯	11E T◯ F◯
12	12A T◯ F◯	12B T◯ F◯	12C T◯ F◯	12D T◯ F◯	12E T◯ F◯
13	13A T◯ F◯	13B T◯ F◯	13C T◯ F◯	13D T◯ F◯	13E T◯ F◯
14	14A T◯ F◯	14B T◯ F◯	14C T◯ F◯	14D T◯ F◯	14E T◯ F◯
15	15A T◯ F◯	15B T◯ F◯	15C T◯ F◯	15D T◯ F◯	15E T◯ F◯
16	16A T◯ F◯	16B T◯ F◯	16C T◯ F◯	16D T◯ F◯	16E T◯ F◯
17	17A T◯ F◯	17B T◯ F◯	17C T◯ F◯	17D T◯ F◯	17E T◯ F◯
18	18A T◯ F◯	18B T◯ F◯	18C T◯ F◯	18D T◯ F◯	18E T◯ F◯
19	19A T◯ F◯	19B T◯ F◯	19C T◯ F◯	19D T◯ F◯	19E T◯ F◯
20	20A T◯ F◯	20B T◯ F◯	20C T◯ F◯	20D T◯ F◯	20E T◯ F◯
21	21A T◯ F◯	21B T◯ F◯	21C T◯ F◯	21D T◯ F◯	21E T◯ F◯
22	22A T◯ F◯	22B T◯ F◯	22C T◯ F◯	22D T◯ F◯	22E T◯ F◯
23	23A T◯ F◯	23B T◯ F◯	23C T◯ F◯	23D T◯ F◯	23E T◯ F◯
24	24A T◯ F◯	24B T◯ F◯	24C T◯ F◯	24D T◯ F◯	24E T◯ F◯
25	25A T◯ F◯	25B T◯ F◯	25C T◯ F◯	25D T◯ F◯	25E T◯ F◯
26	26A T◯ F◯	26B T◯ F◯	26C T◯ F◯	26D T◯ F◯	26E T◯ F◯
27	27A T◯ F◯	27B T◯ F◯	27C T◯ F◯	27D T◯ F◯	27E T◯ F◯
28	28A T◯ F◯	28B T◯ F◯	28C T◯ F◯	28D T◯ F◯	28E T◯ F◯
29	29A T◯ F◯	29B T◯ F◯	29C T◯ F◯	29D T◯ F◯	29E T◯ F◯
30	30A T◯ F◯	30B T◯ F◯	30C T◯ F◯	30D T◯ F◯	30E T◯ F◯

MCQ
TEST 4

Time allowed – one hour

All questions must be answered by filling in the true/false or don't know boxes on the computer marking sheet

1 *In uncomplicated acute hepatitis, patients should be advised to*

A Follow a strict fat-free diet for 1 month.
B Rest in bed only if they feel unwell.
C Abstain from alcohol for at least 3 months.
D Avoid strenuous physical activity for the duration of jaundice.
E Desist from sexual intercourse for as long as they are potentially infectious.

2 *In the management of severe hypoglycaemia, glucagon*

A Would not be effective if the patient had severe liver disease.
B Must be given by deep subcutaneous injection.
C Increases the blood glucose concentration within 2–3 minutes.
D May be issued to relatives of insulin-treated patients for emergency use.
E Recognized side effects include vomiting.

3 *Persistent hoarseness in an adult*

A Occurs if firm apposition of the vocal cords is prevented.
B For longer than 3 weeks demands urgent laryngoscopy.
C Recognized causes include carcinoma of the bronchus.

D From overuse/abuse, patients should be advised to whisper for a few weeks.
E May be a feature of arthritis.

4 *Enuretic alarms*

A Cannot be used effectively before the age of 7 years.
B Principle involved is aversion therapy.
C Child should sleep naked from the waist down.
D Are obtainable on NHS prescription.
E Cannot be used for deaf children.

5 *Carcinoma of the prostate*

A Initial presenting symptoms include dribbling micturition.
B Gland is enlarged, smooth and mobile on rectal examination.
C Always causes an elevation in serum prostatic acid phosphatase.
D Metastatic disease is present in nearly 50 per cent of patients at diagnosis.
E Treatment of choice is total prostatectomy.

6 *Legionnaire's disease*

A Is caused by a virus.
B Affects men and women equally.
C May present with abdominal pain and diarrhoea.
D Rarely produces cerebral confusion.
E Treatment of choice is tetracycline.

27

7 In a patient on lithium, clinically significant drug interactions may occur with concurrent taking of

A Thiazide diuretics.
B Ibuprofen (Brufen).
C Magnesium trisilicate antacid.
D Aspirin.
E Oral hypoglycaemics.

8 The majority of children with acute otitis media

A Are brought to a GP within 24–36 hours of the onset of pain.
B Have earache at night.
C Will go on to develop glue ear.
D Need 7 days of an appropriate antibiotic for effective treatment.
E Will still have obvious loss of hearing 6 weeks after the attack.

9 Lactation

A If failing, may be stimulated by a short course of metoclopramide (Maxolon).
B Is normally suppressed within 1–2 days of stopping breast feeding.
C After a stillbirth can be suppressed by bromocriptine (Parlodel).
D And the progestogen-only Pill provide almost 100 per cent contraception.
E May transfer lipid- but not water-soluble drugs Mum has taken, to the baby.

10 Longitudinal studies in epidemiology

A Look for associations between a disease and possible aetiological factors.
B Study a group (cohort) of persons more than once.
C Provide prevalence data.
D Are the only practical method of studying rare diseases.
E Can help determine the natural history of a disease.

11 After a stroke

A Some dysphasic patients can still read and write.
B Tricyclic antidepressants would be the drugs of choice for treatment of associated depression.
C Patients should be advised that sexual activity is dangerous.
D Painful hemiplegic shoulder can be prevented by careful nursing in the early stages.
E Day centre attendance is very unlikely to be appropriate.

12 In the treatment of acne, benzoyl peroxide preparations

A Must not be used on recently washed skin.
B Should be put on the entire skin area affected and not just the spots.
C Are only available on prescription.
D Will produce a moderate reddening and peeling of the skin within a few days.
E Should be started at 10 per cent concentration.

13 Acute idiopathic thrombocytopenic purpura

A Typically affects 20- to 50-year-old women.
B Blood count (other than platelets) is normal.
C May follow 1–2 weeks after a (usually) viral infection.
D Presenting symptom may be florid bleeding.
E Will in most cases become chronic and need treatment with steroids.

14 In the NHS, domiciliary visits by consultants

A Are most often made by psychiatrists.
B Average out to about 18 visits per GP per year.
C In 80 per cent of cases are carried out with both GP and consultant present.
D Fee is allowable for visits made at instigation of specialist to review the urgency of a proposed hospital admission.
E Must be to patients who on medical grounds cannot attend hospital.

15 Stress incontinence

A Is urinary leakage accompanied by a strong desire to void.
B Only ever affects women.
C Initial examination may include that of the central nervous system.
D In most patients will be improved by anticholinergic drugs.
E In nearly all cases will be cured by anterior colporrhaphy.

16 *A patient is getting repeated attacks of palpitations. Features suggesting paroxysmal tachycardia rather than anxiety state include*

A Pulse rate well over 140 per minute.
B Sweating during the attack.
C Attacks come on very suddenly.
D Associated fine tremor of the fingers.
E Increased pulse rate does not slow during sleep.

17 *In the treatment of psoriasis, 'short-contact' therapy with dithranol*

A Begins with the 2% strength.
B Is generally applied for 30 minutes each day.
C Cream should be rubbed into lesion and at least a 1-cm ring of normal skin.
D Should not be used on the face.
E If used on the scalp may discolour fair hair brown.

18 *Recognized features of mania include*

A Elated mood.
B Auditory hallucinations.
C Psychomotor retardation.
D Flight of ideas.
E Feelings of passivity.

19 *In children, flat feet*

A Are normal in the neonatal period.
B Are mobile when the medial arch returns when the child stands on tiptoe.
C That are stiff should be referred to hospital.
D Causing excessive shoe wear may be helped by insoles.
E Should be treated with foot exercises and physiotherapy.

20 *A doctor signing a medical certificate of cause of death must*

A Have seen and examined the body after death.
B Deliver the certificate to the registrar personally or by post.
C Be, or be the partner of, the doctor who attended the deceased during the last illness.
D Never use the term 'old age' or 'senility' as a cause of death.
E Not complete a certificate with the mode of dying as the only entry.

21 *Cluster headaches (migrainous headaches)*

A Occur as often in women as in men.
B Pain is characteristically localized behind one eye.
C Symptoms tend to occur for up to 2–3 months at a time.
D Only recognized associated neurological sign is Horner's syndrome.
E May be effectively treated with prophylactic ergotamine.

22 *In the treatment of epilepsy, sodium valproate (Epilim)*

A Major indications include petit mal and grand mal seizures.
B Tablets are best taken on an empty stomach.
C May cause temporary thinning of the hair.
D Plasma concentrations correlate well with anticonvulsant efficacy.
E Patient with vague ill health should have urgent screening of liver function performed.

23 *Helpful advice to give 20- to 50-year-old patients with difficulties getting to sleep includes*

A Do something distracting and absorbing in the hour before bed.
B Try to get to sleep at the same time each night.
C Use an alarm clock to wake at the same time each morning.
D Avoid daytime naps.
E Lack of sleep is not harmful.

24 *Characteristic features of acute glaucoma include*

A Absent red reflex.
B Normal visual acuity.
C Severe ocular pain.
D Constricted pupil.
E Dramatic response to 4% pilocarpine drops.

25 *After the death of an important relative, older children*

A Before the age of 9–10 are unlikely to have any concept of the permanence of death.
B Feelings of grief are almost always accompanied by loss of confidence.

C Should not be allowed to attend the funeral.

D Adjust more rapidly to the loss than adults.

E May feel responsible for the death.

26 Recognized causes of macrocytosis on a blood film report include

A Pregnancy.

B Thalassaemia.

C Alcoholism.

D Marrow infiltration.

E Folate deficiency.

27 In pityriasis rosea

A The herald patch is larger than subsequent lesions.

B Lesions show a peripheral collarette of scale.

C The eruption is symmetrical.

D Topical corticosteroids are contraindicated.

E Natural resolution occurs within 3–4 weeks of onset.

28 Choroiditis (posterior uveitis)

A May be caused by toxoplasmosis.

B Presentation is classically with pain in the eye.

C Visual loss is inevitably progressive.

D Retina will show 'bone-corpuscle' pigment deposits at the periphery.

E Treatment of choice is prednisolone eye drops.

29 Recognized visual developmental milestones include

A Newborn, transient visual fixation on moving face.

B At 6 weeks, recognizes mother and bottle.

C At 6 months, responds quickly to object in peripheral vision.

D At 12 months, watches cars, people, dogs outdoors to about 20 feet.

E At 5 years, develops colour vision.

30 Chorionic villus sampling

A Is carried out at 12–14 weeks.

B Will obtain more tissue than amniocentesis.

C Hazards include an increased abortion rate of 2–3 per cent.

D Technique involves dilating the cervix.

E Is of value as placental tissue contains the same chromosomes and enzymes as the fetus.

THE ANSWERS TO MCQ TEST 4 BEGIN ON PAGE 42

1 A False Pneumococcal by far the commonest. Viral or atypical in 25–40 per cent.

B False Found in less than 25 per cent. Most have inspiratory crackles.

C False Only indicated if recovery is slow.

D False Amoxycillin or erythromycin.

E True Also if after 'flu as deterioration may be very rapid even in previously fit young adults.

2 A True Disulfiram-like reaction.

B True Also increased activity of tolbutamide, warfarin.

C True Also decreased tetracycline absorption if taken with milk or antacids.

D True Other antibiotics may interfere with Pill absorption but rare and difficult to predict.

E False Like penicillins have little in way of interactions.

3 A False From damage or destruction of the hair cells in the cochlea.

B False Tinnitus is from damage to sensorineural part of auditory system.

C False May cause tinnitus. Carbamazepine gives good results but probably few cases in which its use is justified.

D True Often better than maskers alone.

E False Less than 50 per cent of patients likely to benefit.

4 A False Occurs only in the presence of a specific object or situation.

B False Beyond voluntary control.

C False The phobic realizes the irrationality of the fears.

D False From the Greek for market place, this means fear of situations which contain a lot of people.

E True This is the important feature clinically.

5 A True FPC may impose conditions on use.

B True Place or time whether have appointment system or not.

C True If no consent from FPC may appeal to Secretary of State.

D False Although must ensure deputy is eligible for medical list.

E True FPC will consider representations and consult Local Medical Committee (LMC).

6 A False Symmetrical, mainly affecting thighs and shoulders.

B True This and (elevated) ESR are the only investigations likely to help confirm the diagnosis.

C False Nor to paracetamol, while response to prednisolone is dramatic.

D False Natural course from 1 to 10 years or more.

E True Also proximal limb pains.

7 A False Occluded areas of skin most often affected.

B True Start as small erythematous macules with a central minivesicle.

C True Because of large areas of anhidrosis.

D **False** Although cooling solutions such as calamine and measures to combat sweating will help more.

E **True** To decrease sweat production and increase evaporation.

8 A **True** Review patient then to ensure all is OK.

B **False** Firm pad relieves discomfort.

C **False** Routine antibiotic drops need to be applied 2–3 hourly.

D **True** Illegal.

E **False** This mainly applies to vaccines, parenteral drugs and coils.

9 A **False** Up to 50 per cent by HSV-1 from partner's labial cold sores.

B **False** For most is a severe illness with localized genital discomfort, fever and systemic upset.

C **True** If lesions on cervix. Ulcers on vulva and urethra give severe dysuria.

D **True** To prevent autoinoculation need to have good genital hygiene.

E **False** Oral is best; 200 mg five times a day for 5 days.

10 A **True** And have no reason to suppose it is not genuine.

B **True** Also a locked glove compartment whereas the same drugs in a locked bag in a locked car do not comply.

C **False** Although a good habit, is not legally required.

D **True** Each GP's register should be ready for such inspection either by police or the Divisional Medical Officer of the Regional Service of the DHSS.

E **True** Within 7 days of consultation whether prescription given or not.

11 A **False** On a treadmill.

B **False** Graded so can assess weakest to fittest.

C **False** One in 1000 to 1 in 5000 risk of ventricular fibrillation, 1 in 10 000 or so death.

D **True** Although patient may be encouraged to continue a little longer if safe and likely to help diagnosis.

E **True** If marked chest pain is induced by exercise then test will stop.

12 A **True** Or hypothalamic pituitary dysfunction.

B **True** At any time if no recent uterine bleeding otherwise on or about fifth day of cycle.

C **True** If occurs discontinue course and give no further courses.

D **True** And pregnancy rate by 50 per cent.

E **True** About 8 per cent will have twins or more!

13 A **True** Aching pain also aggravated by activity.

B **False** Unreliable sign.

C **True** Also giving way and occasional swelling of knee joint.

D **False** Clinical diagnosis is sufficient.

E **True** Lie down; turn feet slightly outwards; lift heels 4 inches (10 cm) off bed or floor; repeat 500 times per day. In theory prevents patella from subluxing laterally.

14 A **True** Expecially in families with multiple problems

B **False** Normal schoolchildren have an average of four to six bruises.

C **True** Most significant areas are cheeks, jaw, ear or mastoid.

D **True** Can also cause subdural haematoma.

E **False** If suspect take action by informing paediatrician, social services, NSPCC or police. Failure to act endangers child.

15 A **False** Nulliparous or first child after the age of 25.

B **False** Early menarche or late menopause.

C **False** No real evidence of this.

D **True** Or history of cancer in the other breast.

E **True** Especially if mother had bilateral breast disease.

16 A **True** Although only if urine is centrifuged and spun deposit resuspended before microscopy.

B **True** May give rise to transient, less than 48 hours, haematuria.

C **True** At least 20 per cent have serious abnormality (50 per cent malignancy).

D **False** Don't blame the warfarin without further investigation.

E **True** Mostly will have benign, essential haematuria.

17 *A* **True** With hair loss.

B **True** Essentially a childhood infection.

C **False** If fungus is from a human source, inflammation is mild.

D **False** If fungus is from an animal source, e.g. cat or dog, then inflammation is pronounced and may produce a boggy, purulent, painful mass known as a kerion.

E **True** 10 mg/kg body weight daily for 4–6 weeks.

18 *A* **False** School phobic is distressed and anxious.

B **True** Also better behaviour and higher IQ than the truant.

C **True** Overanxious, overprotective mother possibly with neurotic illness.

D **False** Phobics stay at home while truants don't.

E **False** Truant is often antisocial from antisocial background.

19 *A* **False** Twelve weeks then improve spontaneously.

B **False** About two-thirds.

C **False** Most often on first rising.

D **True** In some others treatment of symptoms of oesophageal reflux may help.

E **False** Best advice is to avoid drug therapy but if needed then antihistamine group drug should be used.

20 *A* **True** Abnormal if height falls away from original centile position.

B **False** May be normally tall (tall parents) or normally short (many Asian children).

C **False** Discrepancies between height and weight centiles are often great.

D **True** On average grow 3 cm in this period (more in early years of life and during puberty).

E **True** Fifty per cent of that age group taller; 50 per cent shorter.

21 *A* **True** About two per GP every 3 years.

B **False** Essentially clinical diagnosis. EEG may be normal between fits in 30 per cent of epileptics and abnormal in 20 per cent of non-epileptics.

C **True** Although of all epileptics less than 1 per cent have cerebral tumours.

D **True** Phenytoin once daily; other two to three times.

E **True** Or going to discos as known precipitating factors.

22 *A* **True** Apical – radial deficit in fibrillation makes radial pulse unreliable.

B **False** Leads to increased plasma levels so use reduced dose.

C **True** After 2–3 months.

D **False** Usually a clinical diagnosis confirmed if improvement follows in 3–4 days of reducing/stopping the drug.

E **False** Within 3–4 days.

23 *A* **True** Seventy-five per cent of empty scrotal sacs due to retractile testes.

B **True** Previously impalpable testes may now be detected.

C **True** Can always be manipulated into the lower scrotum.

D **True** Malignancy risks outweigh those of anaesthetic.

E **False** Ideally at 2 but certainly before 5 years.

24 *A* **False** Use within 1 hour or discard.

B **True** If doesn't prevent, may modify.

C **True** With human dilute immunoglobulin to modify any reaction.

D **False** Although might be if was on regular fluorinated steroids and would be if was receiving regular oral steroids.

E **True** Immunity likely to be lifelong if given at 15 months or later.

25 *A* **True** And by the doctor doing the recommendation.

B **False** Seventy-two hours then may need action under different section.

C **False** No right of appeal for the 72 hours.

D **True** Or the section lapses.

E **False** Must be nearest relative, not any relative.

26 A **False** Tend to be elderly, maturity-onset, non-insulin dependent.

B **False** Severely dehydrated but no hyperventilation.

C **True** Very high blood and urine glucose.

D **False** This would suggest hypoglycaemia.

E **False** Tend to be quite sensitive and hospital should use reduced doses compared to ketoacidotic case.

27 A **False** At least 2 hours.

B **False** One thorough lotion treatment should suffice.

C **True** Although should never be relied on.

D **True** Lower toxicity and less insect resistance.

E **False** Good hair care with regular, frequent brushing or combing is excellent preventative.

28 A **True** Pain and swelling come with eating and subside shortly after.

B **False** Only if impacted in or near the orifice of the submandibular duct.

C **True** Pain there also.

D **False** Large majority are radio-opaque.

E **True** If in duct otherwise external approach and gland removed *in toto.*

29 A **False** Two minutes. Better definition is 'couple feel their sex life is being spoiled by the man's too rapid ejaculation'.

B **False** True premature ejaculators are young men with good erections. With loss of erection may be a sign of impotence.

C **True** For example may have too long foreplay.

D **True** Utilizes pain to abolish erectile and ejaculatory response.

E **True** Delays ejaculation in some men and worth trying.

30 A **False** Only while baby is fully breast fed on demand.

B **False** No increase in complications if fitted after the fourth week.

C **True** Refit once pregnancy changes have regressed as far as possible.

D **False** Best if readmit after 6–8 weeks.

E **False** If not breast feeding can straight away.

MCQ
TEST 2

Answers

1 A **False** Peak incidence in 15- to 35-year-old non-smokers

B **True** Stool retention can occur proximal to the inflamed rectum. Most present with tenesmus, loose stools with blood and mucus.

C **True** Often nothing to find except a feeling of warmth on rectal examination caused by the presence of inflammation.

D **True** Steroids of greatest value in acute attacks.

E **False** Lesions are flat or *in situ* so barium enema is inappropriate. Patients at risk should undergo colonoscopy and multiple biopsies at 2-yearly intervals.

2 A **False** Reduces carbohydrate tolerance so increases blood glucose levels.

B **False** Commonly hyponatraemia.

C **True** Particularly in immobile or prostatic patient.

D **True** Although uncommon in old people.

E **False** Decrease it. Hypercalcaemia may occur in patients taking calcium salts, e.g. in antacids.

3 A **True** Or carious.

B **True** If infection spreads round muscles of mastication.

C **False** Mostly sensitive. Add metronidazole if an obvious abscess yields no pus on incision.

D **False** Drainage will give quicker relief to the patient.

E **False** This fee is for arresting a dental haemorrhage or removal of dental plugs or stitches.

4 A **False** 21–24 months for this. At 18 months can say number of words with meaning.

B **False** This should have started at 12 months and be finished now.

C **True** Singly by 2 years.

D **True** And telling Mum that he wants the potty.

E **False** Walking from 13 months but not running until 2 years.

5 A **False** Pain only when ovulation begins to occur regularly.

B **False** Shortly before the flow and passes off in 12–24 hours.

C **False** Very unlikely to be any pelvic lesion and examination may be upsetting.

D **False** Inhibits prostaglandin synthesis – like NSAIDs – so prevents muscle contraction and associated pain.

E **False** If NSAIDs not effective low dose combined Pill will be.

6 A **True** May have pains in back, trunk, limbs made worse by jarring or flexing the spine.

B **False** These are characteristic of osteomalacia.

C **False** This would suggest Paget's disease. In osteoporosis, biochemical investigations are normal.

D **True** From vertebral collapse.

E **True** Characteristic from buckling of the trunk due to kyphosis.

7 A **True** From stimulation of appetite.

B **True** Can cause drowsiness. Also caution regarding machinery, alcohol.

C **True** Up to 3 mg may be given as a single, daily dose.

D **True** Unlike methysergide has no long-term side effects.

E **False** Has powerful antiserotonin and antitryptamine properties.

8 A **True** Protects many patients from relapse. Poor compliers may need depot injections.

B **False** All need some satisfying form of carefully paced activity open to them. Will not tolerate too much stimulation.

C **True** Key figure in home management.

D **True** May also benefit patient if reduces family tensions.

E **False** Ready access needed but not intrusive or dependence inducing care.

9 A **False** Middle-aged manual workers.

B **True** Diagnosis confirmed if pain reproduced by abduction arm against examiner's resisting hand.

C **False** Encourage active movements.

D **True** Better than injecting directly into tendon as may rupture.

E **True** If pain persistent and disabling, division of the coraco-acromial ligament usually gives good result.

10 A **True** Unlike form Med 3.

B **True** So long as there is an adequate written record in the notes.

C **False** Report must be no more than 1 month old.

D **True** In the space provided at the bottom.

E **False** If not in patient's interest give less precise diagnosis and inform DMO of the facts on form Med 6.

11 A **False** Bleeding starts after several hours or days.
B **True** So long as mother has been identified as a carrier.
C **True** All sons normal, all daughters carriers.
D **False** Can only stop bleeding and will not resolve haematomas etc.
E **False** Although should be warned only to have sexual intercourse with a sheath as semen may transmit the virus.

12 A **True** Endemic human parvovirus infection.
B **True** Characteristic 'slapped-cheek' appearance.
C **False** Itch, headache, sore throat, runny nose, sore eyes, stomach ache may precede the rash.
D **True** Both facial and maculopapular (trunk/limbs) rashes last up to 1 week but tend to recur over following weeks.
E **False** May go to school and no specific treatment required.

13 A **False** May be, but usually gradual over few days or weeks.
B **True** Although sometimes patient may smile deceptively.
C **False** Constipation. Also reduced libido.
D **True** Restlessness and early waking.
E **False** Weight loss is usual.

14 A **False** Split usually in posterior midline and maintained by sphincter spasm. Can be demonstrated by eversion of anal margin.
B **False** May persist for long periods after.
C **True** Often occurs
D **False** Bulking agents to soften stool, high fibre diet, local anaesthetic ointment to reduce pain is normal management.
E **True** Or lateral cutaneous sphincterotomy. No evidence that anal dilators are of much value.

15 A **False** 1974 when NHS was reorganized.
B **False** Statutory duties to produce an annual report and to hold an annual meeting with the District Health Authority (DHA)
C **False** Annual budget from the Regional Health Authority.
D **False** Nominees of the local authority, local voluntary bodies and the Regional Health Authority.
E **True** If formal complaint made is forwarded to the district administrator.

16 A **True** Magnetic resonance imaging scans can also help diagnostically.
B **False** Less than 10 per cent seriously disabled in 5 years; 20 per cent work with full social life for 10 years or more.
C **False** Only if previous pregnancy resulted in severe relapse.
D **True** May also reduce nocturnal urinary frequency.
E **False** Nor will it affect the rate of progression of the disease.

17 A **True** So at least 6 weeks for steady-state concentration.
B **True** Remarkably well tolerated.
C **True** Check all patients with active disease for this 2–3 weeks after starting tamoxifen.
D **False** Thirty per cent will respond with a reduction in tumour deposits.
E **True** Also first-line therapy in advanced disease in postmenopausal.

18 A **False** Of recent onset, shows infection spread to involve labyrinth and requires urgent hospital referral.
B **False** Pain is not a feature.
C **True** Usually present.
D **False** Not characteristic but not uncommon and presents as collection of white material either in attic or posterior drum.
E **True** Inspection of the drum shows discharge is from middle ear.

19 *A* **True** Harsh, barking cough and stridor develop gradually.

B **True** Admit if rate more than 60 per minute.

C **False** Viral illness so antibiotics not indicated.

D **False** Two-year-olds in late autumn/early winter.

E **False** May provoke respiratory obstruction. Need warm, humidified air.

20 *A* **True** Nor other drugs which could be hoarded for misuse.

B **True** A patient-held repeat card can help this.

C **False** Mistakes more likely if not written by GP, although of course the signatory is the one who is legally responsible.

D **True** Must dictate when and how often patient to be seen.

E **True** Lists drugs; number of repeats allowed and given etc.

21 *A* **False** Up to 40–45 years after even relatively short exposure.

B **False** Most common symptom and usually persistent and severe.

C **False** Occurs in fewer than 10 per cent of patients.

D **True** No cure and treatment essentially palliative.

E **True** Also cough and sometimes haemoptysis as disease advances.

22 *A* **False** Most often adult males after middle age.

B **False** Symptomless enlargement which only rarely gives rise to obstruction.

C **True** Unlike rosacea.

D **False** Have little effect although may help if patient has a lot of pustules.

E **True** Or surgical shaving of the affected areas.

23 *A* **False** Young men in their sexual prime.

B **True** Mostly married Caucasians with sociopathic traits.

C **True** Will masturbate at the time or use as fantasy material for future.

D **True** And more likely to reoffend and show no remorse.

E **True** Or imprisoned for 3 months; 80 per cent of those who appear before the courts do not reoffend.

24 *A* **True** Prime site of action. Also affects cervical mucus, tubal motility, ovulation.

B **False** No resistance to contraceptive effect with time.

C **False** About 4 hours so get maximum effect on cervical mucus.

D **False** Contraindications different from those of the combined Pill.

E **False** No evidence that this is necessary.

25 *A* **True** Age prevalence is one of increasing with age.

B **True** Of those diagnosed 50 per cent are being treated and in 50 per cent of them the raised blood pressure is controlled.

C **False** Fifty per cent are over 60 when first diagnosed.

D **True** Is hypertension worth treating in the over 60s?

E **False** Major risk is death from stroke.

26 *A* **True** In women, is age in years + 10 divided by 2.

B **True** Do this by affecting serum proteins.

C **True** Also if smoking, obesity, pregnancy or on the Pill.

D **False** Simple, cheap investigation, easily performed in treatment room by GP or practice nurse.

E **True** Malignancy, myelomatosis, renal disease, subacute bacterial endocarditis, tuberculosis are all causes.

27 *A* **False** Taken at all ages, including babies and during pregnancy.

B **False** One or two doses prior to exposure helps confirm tolerance and allows time for adequate blood levels to develop.

C **False** No drug combination can be relied on to be 100 per cent effective.

D **True** At least four and preferably six.

E **True** Private prescription. Chloroquine and proguanil can be bought without prescription.

28 *A* **True** Although may be diffuse or even bilateral.

B **True** Not from the ectopic site but from the breakdown of the decidual lining of the uterus.

C **False** Gravindex of little help in reaching diagnosis unlike ultrasound and laparoscopy.

D **False** Although pulse rate is normally raised.

E **False** This and faintness each occur in about 10–15 per cent of cases.

29 *A* **True** Once tear production has begun.

B **True** From proximal to the obstruction.

C **False** Unless sticky eye in first few days of life when must make sure is not chlamydial or gonococcal infection.

D **False** No risk to eye even from most unpleasant looking mucopus.

E **True** If not, then probing of the duct will be necessary.

30 *A* **True** Three to six months after gluten-containing foods come into diet.

B **True** Or pass frequent pale, bulky, offensive stools.

C **False** Miserable, apathetic, pale with abdominal distension.

D **True** And sometimes oats.

E **False** Patient much better within days but this takes up to 1 year.

MCQ
TEST 3

Answers

1 *A* **False** Twenty- to thirty-year-olds; 13 men to 1 woman sex ratio.

B **True** Reiter's syndrome appears to be a specific host response in genetically predisposed individuals.

C **False** Seronegative arthritis follows a few days after urethritis.

D **False** By conjunctivitis.

E **True** Occurs in 25 per cent of male patients and usually heals spontaneously.

2 *A* **True** Caused by altered peripheral vascular permeability and relatively resistant to diuretics.

B **True** Also headache, flushing from the vasodilatation.

C **False** Does not seem to adversely affect lipids or uric acid.

D **True** Reflex tachycardia may do this and in many angina patients needs to be combined with a beta-blocker.

E **True** Also weakness, nausea, insomnia.

3 *A* **True** Nearly all between 5 to 9 years old.

B **True** Deafness noted by either school or parents.

C **False** Conductive deafness usually of 30–40 decibels.

D **True** Yellow, retracted or with air–fluid level.

E **False** Permanent deafness is not a risk and naturally resolves over a few years.

4 *A* **False** Discharged at about 5 days postop.

B **False** A suitable bulky stool will help to prevent stricture.

C **True** From sepsis and will lead to readmission.

D **False** Usually about the same and preoperative reassurance by the GP can be helpful.

E **True** Usually elderly.

5 A **False** Control by taking Pill continuously or possibly by change of progestogen.
  B **True** Stop Pill at once.
  C **True** And should not take again until liver function tests have returned to normal.
  D **False** Although must take additional precautions for rest of that cycle.
  E **False** Not a contraindication.

6 A **True** Burning sensation often radiating to the back of the jaw or between the shoulders.
  B **False** Although can occur occasionally.
  C **False** Worsened by meals and sometimes on stooping or lying flat.
  D **False** Hot drinks may give pain if reflux oesophagitis is present.
  E **False** Implies dysphagia.

7 A **False** Best 1 or 2 hours before symptoms are expected to develop.
  B **True** Paradoxical effect, probably due to its anticholinergic properties.
  C **False** Remarkably free from the serious side effects associated with other phenothiazines.
  D **False** Lower initial doses and more gradual increases in the elderly.
  E **True** Adequate lighting, reduced noise, presence of familiar relative.

8 A **False** To ultraviolet light; similar in pathology to snow blindness.
  B **False** Interval of 6–8 hours before develops.
  C **False** Intense lacrimation, blepharospasm, photophobia in a very miserable patient.
  D **True** Innumerable lesions which heal within a few hours.
  E **False** Need this before can examine the eyes. Relieves the blepharospasm and is usually the only treatment needed.

9 A **True** Affects boys and girls equally.
  B **True** Although in 60 per cent only the legs – either the shins or deep in the thighs or calves.
  C **False** Only 25 per cent at night although can wake child.

  D **False** No signs.
  E **True** The odd paracetamol is unlikely to do any harm.

10 A **False** Suspect cervical spondylosis or carpal tunnel syndrome.
   B **True** May only be referred pain and no pain in the elbow.
   C **True** Also pain aggravated by gripping and twisting.
   D **False** X-ray nearly always normal and diagnosis is clinical.
   E **True** Gives many relief but often recurs so 60 per cent of patients will have symptoms for a year or more.

11 A **False** About 70 per cent cases from disease of the biliary tract.
   B **False** Useful to identify disease but level has no relation to severity or prognosis.
   C **False** Tenderness, rigidity and signs of peritoneal irritation.
   D **False** Pain relief often a problem and may well need opiates.
   E **False** Surgery only if diagnostic doubt or if biliary tract disease needs urgent treatment.

12 A **True** Dose–response relationship for warfarin is steep so even minor interactions may increase risk of bleeding.
   B **True** As can paracetamol.
   C **True** So increasing anticoagulant action.
   D **True** Unlike cimetidine (Tagamet), has no effect on warfarin action.
   E **True** Oestrogens will antagonize the effect of warfarin.

13 A **True** Insidious onset with lethargy, deterioration in mood and difficulty in coping.
   B **True** May stem from concern for her own health or that of her baby.
   C **False** No definite predisposing factors yet known.
   D **False** Treatment of choice with psychotherapy and practical support from family, friends etc.
   E **False** This would suggest a much more severe psychosis and only occurs rarely.

14 A False No significant correlation with road accidents.
 B False Unless getting side effects like vertigo, dizziness, faintness or postural hypotension.
 C True However well controlled may seem to be.
 D False No fit since the age of 5 years.
 E True As with any progressive or disabling disorder of the nervous system.

15 A True Or lichen simplex et atrophicus.
 B False Occur in the elderly.
 C False Painless lump or ulcer which gradually enlarges. May cause pain, itching or bleeding in some patients.
 D False Vulvectomy with block dissection of affected glands.
 E False Prognosis depends on metastasis which is difficult to detect.

16 A True Once detectable titre rises rapidly with doubling time of 12–24 hours.
 B False Isolation of the virus has no place in the diagnosis of rubella as it is so unreliable.
 C False Take further serum as soon as possible – if the titre is rising then is recent rubella; if same then infection was in remote past.
 D True Patient immune at time of stated contact.
 E False Not cost effective because high percentage of seroconversion after immunization.

17 A False Minor cold injury often seen in outdoors sportspeople.
 B False Are itchy and may become secondarily infected.
 C True Mauve swollen patches especially on young women who ride horses.
 D False Mauve.
 E False Caused by local rewarming before tissue metabolic demands can be adequately met because of vasoconstriction. Warm body before affected part.

18 A False Only about 15 per cent are in the normal range.

 B True In almost all cases leads to lifelong handicap.
 C True Non-verbal as well as verbal (half are mute).
 D False Characteristically poor sleep, temper tantrums, screaming, overactivity and destructiveness.
 E False Pattern of behaviour produced by wide variety of causes of brain damage or dysfunction, e.g. maternal rubella, perinatal anoxia.

19 A False Most often in primigravid patients.
 B True Hypertension (diastolic 90 mmHg or above) is the central sign.
 C False Usually slowly progressive and only 1–2 per cent of cases will become fulminating.
 D True Also if history of hypertension or renal disease; multiple pregnancy or hydatidiform mole.
 E False Asymptomatic unless fulminating.

20 A True Or in connection with their bodily functions.
 B True Can claim before 6 months if clear need will persist.
 C False Nor for patients in hospital.
 D True About £10 more per week.
 E False Lower limit of 2 years, no upper limit.

21 A False All permanently catheterized patients will develop bacteriuria and no point treating unless a systemic infection.
 B False If small less reaction; 12–14 best if urine clear.
 C False Frequent emptying more comfortable and reduces pressure from a heavy, hanging bag.
 D True More will not stop patient pulling it out, but will increase urethral damage.
 E False Change if stops draining or at most 3 monthly.

22 A True Often with dramatic intensity.
 B False Side effects are not uncommon and may be severe.

C **True** Also more effective in anxious individuals and possibly those of lower intelligence.

D **True** Most desirable effect which can make ineffective remedies effective and increase the benefit from active drugs.

E **True** New remedies can be compared with established placebo treatment.

23 *A* **False** Family history in less than 5 per cent.

B **True** Deafness and tinnitus increase during episodes of vertigo with improvement after.

C **False** *See* answer (B).

D **True** Then number of bilateral cases increases gradually.

E **False** May have sensation pressure in ears but fully conscious.

24 *A* **False** Up to 90 per cent.

B **False** Best interest of child must be put before needs and wishes of the adult.

C **False** Children are not natural liars. False retraction under family pressure is far commoner than false allegation.

D **True** Need full range swabs and careful examination.

E **True** All may contribute pieces to the jigsaw.

25 *A* **False** Also not necessary if employed less than 16 hours per week.

B **False** Outside working hours.

C **True** Irrespective of how long she has been employed.

D **False** Terms of service vary from practice to practice.

E **True** Showing gross wages, what deductions, net pay.

26 *A* **False** Past 8–12 weeks.

B **False** 10–12 per cent moderately good, over 15 per cent unacceptable.

C **False** Value not affected by recent food intake.

D **True** As in haemolytic anaemia.

E **False** Prolonged periods of hypoglycaemia, e.g. at night, may lower value to normal range.

27 *A* **True** Widespread bilateral symmetrical itch which does not involve the head, centre of chest or centre of back then *is* scabies.

B **True** Overwhelming majority of mites are on the hands.

C **True** Viable mites never leave the body and cannot survive if they do.

D **True** Latter is very uncomfortable to patients with excoriated skin.

E **False** Not scientifically based and probably counterproductive.

28 *A* **True** Or active preparations made, e.g. saving up tablets.

B **True** Or precautions taken to avoid discovery.

C **True** Making a will/organizing insurance.

D **False** Heavy drinking so often involved is of little predictive value.

E **True** Or failing to alert helpers during or after the attempt.

29 *A* **False** No special weight to reach and vaccinate at usual time.

B **False** Good reason to immunize as early as possible to protect a vulnerable child.

C **False** As answer (B)

D **False** If has an acute febrile illness then postpone.

E **False** History of epilepsy in parents or siblings is a relative contraindication to pertussis vaccination.

30 *A* **False** Half pint beer or cider; 1 glass wine/sherry; 1 measure spirits.

B **False** For medical practitioners is three times the national average.

C **True** And raised serum gamma-glutamyl transpeptidase.

D **True** As are 42 per cent of patients with serious head injuries.

E **False** About 30–40 with drink problems and 7–10 who are physically dependent on alcohol.

1 A False Reducing fat may help if nausea is a problem.

B True Otherwise bed rest not indicated.

C False Might advise moderation during this time.

D True Although patient feels better as jaundice appears.

E False Use of sheaths will reduce the risk of contamination of mucosal surfaces.

2 A True As acts by mobilizing glycogen stored in the liver.

B False Intramuscular, subcutaneous or intravenous so very useful if patient violent or fitting.

C False Takes 5–20 minutes and if hasn't worked either repeat dose or give intravenous glucose.

D True Useful if patient is prone to hypoglycaemic attacks (hypos).

E True Also nausea and, rarely, hypersensitivity reactions.

3 A True Changes in vocal cord lubrication may also give hoarseness.

B True To exclude a neoplastic cause.

C True At left hilum may paralyse left recurrent laryngeal nerve.

D False Must rest voice. Whispering may strain as much as shouting.

E True Arthritic changes at crico-arytenoid joint will give rise to hoarseness.

4 A False May start at 5 though is more effective over 7 years.

B False Is conditioned learning.

C True So first drop of urine triggers the alarm.

D False Available on loan from Community Health Services in most districts.

E False Silent wakeners which vibrate are good for deaf or where important not to disturb other sleepers.

5 A True Usually identical to those of benign hyperplasia. Anaemia, weight loss and pain from metastases comes later.

B False Hard, nodular and often fixed.

C False Usually elevated if metastases present.

D True Though only 12–15 per cent have symptoms from them and often remain asymptomatic for long periods.

E False Radiotherapy and variety of hormone therapies would be preferred in large majority of cases.

6 A False Short Gram-negative rod bacterium, *Legionella pneumophila*.

B False Rare in children and three times more common in men.

C True Common early symptoms and may dominate clinical picture.

D False Symptoms much the same as other lobar pneumonias but cerebral confusion is very common even in milder cases.

E False Erythromycin.

7 A True May need dose of lithium reduced 25–50 per cent. A loop diuretic should be used in preference to a thiazide.

B True Most NSAIDs reduce lithium excretion.

C True Any medicine with a high sodium content, e.g. Gaviscon, Fybogel, can increase lithium excretion.

D False Has no effect.

E False Safe.

8 A True When signs may be minimal and symptom severity will determine treatment approach.

B True Night cough also common accompanying symptom.

C False Large majority recover without any sequelae.

D **False** Three days is as effective as 7.
E **False** In the large majority, hearing is back to normal in 2–3 weeks.

9 *A* **True** Increase prolactin secretion but only successful if accompanied by suckling.
B **False** Four days.
C **True** 2.5 mg twice daily for 3 weeks. Expensive so not for routine use.
D **True** Progestogen virtually undetectable in the milk.
E **True** Non-protein-bound portion can be transferred by passive diffusion.

10 *A* **True** As do case-control and cross-sectional studies.
B **True** And incidence of disease and changes in the possible aetiological factor determined.
C **False** Cross-sectional study does that.
D **False** Case-control studies for rare disease.
E **True** Also can study the temporal relationship between a possible aetiological factor and the disease.

11 *A* **True** Do not overlook this method of communication.
B **False** Very toxic if brain damage. Mianserin or dothiepin probably better.
C **False** Do not feel too inhibited to mention this aspect of rehabilitation.
D **True** Avoid traction on hemiplegic arm when sitting patient up.
E **False** Particularly useful for taking strain off close carer.

12 *A* **False** Efficacy enhanced if applied after soap and water.
B **True** Once daily for 1–2 weeks then up to twice daily.
C **False** May even be cheaper over the counter.
D **True** Not an indication for stopping.
E **False** Five per cent then 10 or 2.5 per cent depending on response.

13 *A* **False** Mainly 2- to 9-year-olds. Chronic idiopathic thrombocytopenic purpura which is less severe usually affects adults.

B **True** Unless there has been serious blood loss. Platelet count is less than 30×10^9/litre.
C **True** With rapid-onset symptoms.
D **True** Also petechial haemorrhages and purpura.
E **False** Eight per cent spontaneously recover within 6 weeks; 10 per cent become chronic and may need steroids.

14 *A* **False** Geriatricians 217 each per year, psychiatrists 91.
B **True** About 37 per consultant.
C **False** In 50 per cent of cases, both are present at the visit.
D **False** Nor to supervise treatment initiated at hospital.
E **True** Key part of the official definition.

15 *A* **False** This is urge incontinence. In stress, urine is expelled on coughing or straining.
B **False** May follow sphincter damage in prostatectomy.
C **True** For possible early neurological conditions, such as multiple sclerosis.
D **False** Used to decrease detrusor activity in patients with bladder instability.
E **False** Vaginal repair success rate of 50–60 per cent; colposuspension 90 per cent.

16 *A* **True** Usually lower than this in anxiety.
B **False** Sweating, pallor, faintness found in both conditions.
C **True** And without any reason.
D **False** Fine tremor suggests thyrotoxicosis.
E **False** Differentiates thyrotoxicosis from anxiety.

17 *A* **False** Start at 0.1–0.4% and increase strength weekly unless burning occurs.
B **True** Whenever suits patient. Washed off after the 30 minutes.
C **False** Lesions only. May protect normal skin with petroleum jelly.
D **True** Also best avoided in flexures.
E **True** May also discolour skin, clothes, bath.

18 A **True**   Elated, although unstable.
   B **True**   Usually transitory, occurring at the height of the illness.
   C **False** Restless with increased activity.
   D **True**   And over-talkativeness.
   E **False** This is a first rank schizophrenic symptom.

19 A **True**   Medial arch develops fully when walking is established.
   B **True**   Of mobile flat feet 90–95 per cent resolve spontaneously.
   C **True**   Refer rare cases that are symptomatic, stiff, weak or excessively mobile.
   D **True**   Only help the shoe wear, do not 'cure' the feet.
   E **False** Unless there are associated neuromuscular abnormalities, no treatment is required.

20 A **False** Must do this before can sign cremation certificate.
   B **False** May do or can get qualified informant to take it to the registrar.
   C **False** No-one other than the actual attending doctor may sign.
   D **False** If over 70 and no specific condition identified as patient gradually fails then can say died of old age.
   E **True**   Must put down the disease, injury or complication which caused death.

21 A **False** Far commoner in men in whom investigation is not usually indicated.
   B **True**   Severe lasting up to 1–2 hours once or twice a day.
   C **True**   Then often many months before next cluster of attacks.
   D **True**   May occur ipsilateral to symptomatic side of head.
   E **False** Try pizotifen (Sanomigran) or if it fails possibly methysergide (Deseril)–NB with great care.

22 A **True**   Also myoclonic and partial seizures.
   B **False** Immediately after meals to decrease gastrointestinal side effects.
   C **True**   In about 10 per cent of patients.

   D **False** Poorly, although severe side effects more likely if steady state concentration exceeds 10 mg/l.
   E **True**   Especially in first 6 months of therapy as may have idiosyncratic hepatotoxicity.

23 A **True**   To encourage relaxation.
   B **False** Do not go to bed until sleepiness occurs, however late this may be.
   C **True**   Trains natural sleep–waking rhythm. No lie-ins.
   D **True**   Unlike in the elderly where short naps are helpful, in the young they weaken the sleep drive at night.
   E **True**   Most sleep-onset insomniacs take less than 30 minutes to get to sleep.

24 A **True**   With oval, fixed, mid-dilated pupil.
   B **False** Blurred, poor vision.
   C **True**   With headache and vomiting.
   D **False** *See* answer (B). Also may be relative afferent pupil defect in comparison with the other eye.
   E **False** Iris usually too ischaemic to respond. Admit to hospital.

25 A **True**   Although death of pets may have given some idea.
   B **True**   With time adjust to the loss.
   C **False** Should be allowed and even encouraged to share the family grieving.
   D **True**   And the adults may then feel the child is callous.
   E **True**   Children often blame themselves for bad happenings in their lives.

26 A **False** Dilutional effect causes normochromic anaemia.
   B **False** Microcytic, hypochromic anaemia.
   C **True**   Also hypothyroidism, myelodysplastic syndromes.
   D **False** Leucoerythroblastic picture on peripheral film.
   E **True**   Also vitamin B_{12} deficiency or liver disease.

27 **A True** Almost always on the trunk.
  B True And are oval and pink.
  C True On trunk, neck, upper limbs and thighs.
  D False If lot of irritation present, will help suppress it.
  E False Lasts from 6 to 12 weeks.

28 **A True** Although usually no cause found.
  B False Painless floaters, blurred or dim vision and blind spots.
  C False Visual loss due to vitreous exudation during acute attack is usually stationary after.
  D False Retinitis pigmentosa would. See exposed white sclera, exudation, scarring.
  E False May try systemic steroids, immunosuppressives if bad enough.

29 **A True** Also protective blink reflex (to changes in light intensity).

  B False At 6 weeks will follow mother's face. At 3 months recognizes mother and bottle and has hand regard.
  C True Visually alert and can concentrate on new objects for a long time.
  D True Has increasing near and distant acuity.
  E False At 3 years should be able to match two or three colours.

30 **A False** 9–11 weeks so result early enough for vaginal termination of pregnancy if that is necessary.
  B True May be enough cells to make culture unnecessary.
  C True Rate similar to that of amniocentesis.
  D False Small cannula passed through undilated cervix into the placenta.
  E True So a placental biopsy gives same information as cells grown from liquor.

Modified Essay Question or MEQ

The MEQ has become widely used in both undergraduate and postgraduate teaching and most potential MRCGP examinees will have had some experience of the method during their vocational training. As an examination method, it presents particular difficulties, both to candidates and examiners, but because it is capable of sampling a wide range of knowledge, skills and attitudes exhibited by the candidate, it has found a permanent place in the MRCGP examination.

The paper is presented in the form of a booklet, in which each page represents a further development in an unfolding saga. At each stage, additional information is supplied and the candidate is asked to respond to the new situation. In this way the important dimension of time can be built into the story. Because of its open-ended format, the MEQ is extremely flexible and may be used to test much more than factual recall, which is better assessed by the MCQ anyway.

The MEQ may be used to explore the candidates' sensitivity to, and awareness of, the modifying influence of emotional, social and cultural factors in both doctor, patient and society. This point will become clearer as you work through the examples provided. It will be seen that these aspects of the MEQ have become increasingly important and this paper now demands considerable understanding of psychology, sociology and human behaviour if it is to be tackled successfully. It is particularly important to be aware of the considerable complexities inherent in the consultation in general practice.

The questions are deliberately composed in a way which forces the generation of a range of options and an assessment of the advantages and disadvantages of each before a definite decision is taken. The wealth of options offered, and the sensitivity and selectivity demonstrated by the candidate, are what the examiners are looking for. A single option answer, even if technically 'correct', is most unlikely to score high marks by itself. The usual format at present is to set a paper of eight questions and allow the candidate one and a half hours to answer it.

Construction and marking

The construction and marking of an MEQ paper is an extremely time-consuming and complex task if the technique is to remain both valid and reliable. Members of the MEQ group submit outline papers, which are usually based on real cases, to the nucleus group of four examiners under the chairmanship of the MEQ convenor. This group chooses a paper, edits it and then circulates it to the 60 or so examiners who constitute the MEQ group. These examiners then answers the paper as 'examinees' and it is this pool of expertise which forms the basis of the answers.

Groups of eight examiners are each assigned a particular question which becomes their total responsibility. They create a marking schedule by discussion, taking account of the examiners' responses, clarifying any doubtful points by reference to the literature and placing appropriate weight and emphasis on those aspects which the MEQ is most appropriate to assess. They then carry out a trial marking exercise to test the schedule and calibrate their own reliability in using it, because each 'octet' will be responsible for marking its 'own' question in the examination.

A fundamental point to understand is that each question is marked separately and thus every question must be answered in detail on the page on which it is posed. Answer each question specifically even if it means repeating information which you have provided as part of an earlier answer.

The prevailing philosophy of the MEQ group is to encourage markers to recognize the candidate's grasp of concepts rather than worry too much about detailed items in the marking schedule. For this reason, our suggested answers to the examples provided are arranged conceptually.

Technique

As in any examination, knowledge of appropriate technique will help a candidate to maximize his or her potential score and ensure that no marks are lost unnecessarily. It is essential to read the instructions carefully and take notice of them. It is best to present your answers as short notes or lists because this is quicker for you to write and easier for the examiners to mark. Do not read through the paper before you start and do not go back through it afterwards, otherwise the natural progression of the case may be altered and you may be led astray. Most of the questions carry a similar proportion of the marks so try to work steadily through the paper without spending too long on any single section. You are usually informed when you are approximately half-way through the paper.

In this chapter you are provided with four complete MEQs and are allowed one and a half hours to complete each of them. You should try to work under examination conditions, allowing the appropriate time. Do not aim to complete more than one MEQ at a sitting. Do not be surprised if at first you run out of time before finishing. It is difficult to be precise about pass marks but, as a general indication, you should assume that 55 per cent or more represents a comfortable pass, while 40 per cent or less spells probable failure.

The first two papers were actually set in the MRCGP examination within the last few years and, as such, represent the 'state of the art'. We have provided extensive advice and comment as to how we think you should approach these papers and we hope you will find this helpful. We have also suggested some written material which we think would provide useful background information. The marking schedules are intended to give an indication of the range and depth of answers expected. They are flexible enough to allow credit to be given for any reasonable point which we have omitted, but, wherever possible, this should be judged by an independent assessor – possibly a friend, colleague, trainer or course-organizer – rather than by the candidate.

It is an excellent educational exercise to derive group consensus answers to use as a marking schedule. In our experience most group answers will approach 100 per cent while most individuals will find 60 per cent difficult to achieve. Papers three and four provide further practice in answering MEQs without any specific advice or guidance.

Instructions

1 There are eight or nine questions in this and in the subsequent three MEQ papers.
2 Answers should be legible and concise. Total time allowed is **one hour and thirty minutes** per test.
3 Answers should be written in the space provided. If more room is required use the reverse side of the question sheet.
4 You are advised not to alter your answers after completing the whole MEQ and not to look through the book before you start. This may destroy your natural assessment of the case and cause you to lose marks.
5 The MEQ is a test of your practical approach to a developing general practice problem and as such you will gain more marks for your management of the problem than for pure factual knowledge.
6 The available marks may vary between one question and another; you are advised to work steadily through and not delay too long on any one question.
7 Each page of the MEQ is marked independently. You should therefore answer each question specifically, even if this involves repetition of part of an earlier answer.
8 As a rough guide, it is indicated when you are approximately half-way through this paper.

MEQ
TEST 1

The MEQ set in October, 1986 was, in many ways, a classic of the genre. As such, we hope that it will prove a helpful introduction to the present style and content of the MEQ and the expectations of the examiners. We must emphasize that the suggested answers are in no way the 'official' marking schedules, but they should give some guidance as to the priorities which the examiners would emphasize within the range of possible responses.

For the first time in the MEQ, candidates were presented with a past history and problem summary card to read before answering the paper. This is reproduced below:

Surname: SMITH   Forename: Rita   dob 6/10/60   Sex: F

		Height:	5 ft 3 in
1966	T's and A's	Ideal wt	9 stone
1973	Father died myocardial infarct, aged 40 years	Year	1986
1973	School absenteeism	Wt	10.7
1978	Investigated for abdominal pain – no pathology	BP	120/70
1979	Married Robert, Merchant Seaman	Urine	NAD
	(Registered here)	Cx smear	√ 1985
1979	Dizzy spells and palpitations	Alc.	Nil
1980	Headaches, negative investigation	Tob.	Nil
6.1.80	Debbie born. Hyperemesis, forceps	Breast	√ 1985
1984–85	Many unexplained symptoms		

ALLERGIC TO PENICILLIN

Personal and family profile:

Rubella immune 1980
Tetanus toxoid booster Aug. 1986

First, read the past history and problem sheet very carefully. There is an enormous amount of information contained within it.

We get a picture of a slightly overweight lady who has been comprehensively screened and immunized by your recently retired partner. She is allergic to penicillin and has a family history of cardiovascular disease occurring at an early age.

However, what may be more significant is her recurrent presentation of a variety of symptoms for which no organic cause could be found, and which predated her marriage. She also had a difficult pregnancy and delivery 6 years ago.

Before your next patient enters you look at her problem card (*see* page 51), created by your recently retired partner, whose patient she has been. She has not seen you before.

When Mrs Smith comes in she complains of generalized weakness for which you can find no cause. In the course of the consultation, you elicit that she is worried because her Merchant Seaman husband seems obsessed with the belief that he might have AIDS. She asks if he has consulted you recently.

1   What would you wish to cover in the ensuing discussion?

It is best to lay out your answer as a series of points to be covered, headings and subheadings, because this is easier for the examiner to comprehend and quicker for you to write. Remember to think in physical, psychological and social terms and pay attention to management and ethical issues.

Some weeks later Mrs Smith attends complaining of pins and needles in her hands and feet. On full examination you can find no abnormality, and the history together with your previous investigations confirms your impression that this is not an organic disorder.

2   (a) Speculate about the origins of this patient's symptoms.

    (b) How can you help her?

Review all the information you have gained about this patient so far. Consider her past experiences and her present situation. Could there nevertheless be a possible organic cause underlying these symptoms, if so, what might it be? What can you offer her? What options do you have ? Always try and think of yourself in the real clinical situation and how you would respond.

The consultation ends unsatisfactorily. The following day Mr Smith calls to see you, demanding an explanation of his wife's symptoms. He tells you he has made arrangements for her to see a homoeopathic practitioner.

3   *In what ways might you respond?*
    What are the pros and cons of each?

This is a common type of question in the MEQ. You are encouraged to range widely and think laterally! Remember to include all the possible responses, not just those of which you approve. This type of question tests your awareness of the possible implications of any given course of action.

Six months later Mrs Smith complains of loss of vision in one eye. She sees your partner, who suspects she has retrobulbar neuritis, and refers her to a neurologist. The diagnosis of multiple sclerosis is confirmed by his clinical examination and supported by sensory, visual and auditory evoked responses. Later Mr and Mrs Smith come to see you to discuss the neurologist's report.

4 *List the areas you would wish to consider with them at this consultation.*

Unfortunately, neurotic patients are no less likely to develop organic disease than other people, and it can often be difficult to see the wood for the trees. Nevertheless, we all feel upset at missing a significant diagnosis and the important point is whether we react to this guilt constructively or defensively. In addition, we have to consider what the future holds for Mrs Smith, what impact the disease might have on herself and her family, and what we could do to help.

YOU HAVE NOW COMPLETED APPROXIMATELY ONE-HALF
OF THE PAPER

Some time later Mrs Smith brings Debbie, now aged 6, because of a vaginal discharge. She (Debbie) has recently started wetting the bed again and is off her food.

5   (a) *List the possible causes of this presentation.*

     (b) *Outline how you would manage this consultation.*

Part (a) asks you to list the possible causes of this presentation, so do just that. Do not waste time elaborating on your answer. Remember physical, psychological and social causes.

In part (b) try to imagine how you would attempt to structure such a consultation before embarking on further history, examination, investigation and management as appropriate.

Two days later Debbie's schoolteacher phones you in distress. She tells you that Debbie has implied that her father has interfered with her in some way.

6 *What problems does this pose for a GP? How would you deal with them?*

This is a difficult and complex situation, producing a multitude of problems for your contemplation. The child herself, her family and other properly involved authorities must all be taken into consideration as well as your own position. What resources are available to help you deal with this type of problem?

Mr Smith deserts his family and returns to sea. A few days later, Mrs Smith comes to see you. She implies that you have been responsible, to some extent, for the break-up of her marriage. She asks to see her notes to ensure that there is no information recorded which might prejudice her future doctors against her, as she intends to change.

7 *Discuss the different ways in which you might cope with this request to see her notes and the probable consequences of these.*

Again it is most important to note that you are asked to give a range of options, not to select the one which you might choose. The point of this type of question is to see whether you can range widely and consider carefully the pros and cons of any action which you might take. After all, this is much more valuable than exhibiting a conditioned reflex, which is most unlikely to be appropriate to all similar situations.

After consideration, Mrs Smith remains on your list. At 11 p.m. one Saturday evening you receive a telephone call from an anxious neighbour of the Smith family who has been alerted by Debbie knocking on her door. Apparently Mrs Smith is unconscious from an overdose of an antidepressant you had prescribed. You arrange admission to hospital and appropriate care for Debbie.

The following morning you telephone the hospital and discover that Mrs Smith has died.

8 *Describe the thoughts and feelings you might have at this time and the ways you could cope with them.*

The ability and understanding to recognize your own feelings, and make use of them creatively in your professional relationship with patients, is an important attribute for all doctors to cultivate. An honest appraisal of the range of emotions likely to be occasioned by such an event, and a note as to why these are likely to arise, will score high marks. In addition, you must be aware of the support systems which are, or should be, available in order to help you to cope with the inevitable stresses and strains of practice.

THE ANSWERS TO MEQ TEST 1 APPEAR ON PAGE 87

MEQ
TEST 2

Mrs Drummond-Brown, the 47-year-old wife of a senior company executive, presents at your evening surgery without an appointment and demands to be seen straight away. Her manner is so overbearing that she reduces your receptionist to tears. You see her later that session when she greets you with a smile and complains of hot flushes, night sweats and depression.

1 (a) *What reasons can you suggest for the differing ways in which she has presented to you and to your receptionist?*

(b) *What, if anything, might you say to her about the earlier episode in reception?*

Questions dealing with problems of employed and attached staff are not uncommon. You should read *Towards better Practice* (by P. Martin, A. J. Moulds and P. J. Kerrigan, Churchill Livingstone, Edinburgh, 1985) and *Running a Practice: A Manual of Practice Management* (3rd edn, by R. V. Jones, K. J. Bolden, D. J. Gray and M. S. Hall, Methuen, London, 1985), in addition to books on the doctor–patient relationship, such as *The Doctor–Patient Relationship* (3rd edn, by P. Freeling and C. L. Harris, Churchill Livingstone, Edinburgh, 1983) and, of course, the classic by Balint, *The Doctor, his Patient and the Illness* (see book list).

Games People Play by Eric Berne (see book list) is also interesting and informative.

You establish that she is depressed and that the hot flushes are not of sufficient severity to interfere with her way of life.

2   *List the past and present social factors which might have predisposed her to depression?*

You should be familiar with common psychiatric problems because they are such an important feature of general practice. The questions prompt you to consider past and present social factors underlying both endogenous and reactive depression. *Psychiatric Illness in General Practice* (1981, 2nd edn, by Michael Shepherd and Anthony Clare, Oxford University Press, Oxford) and *Psychological Disorders in General Practice* (1979, by P. Williams and A. Clare, Academic Press, London) provide interesting background reading.

Two months later she again comes to your surgery and insists that you prescribe hormone replacement therapy.

3 *What would you want to know before deciding to respond to her request?*

Note the word 'insists'. What does that imply and how would it alter your approach to the consultation. Remember to consider the patient's ideas, concerns and expectations before embarking on the doctor-centred part of the consultation. *Doctors Talking to Patients* (1984, by P. S. Byrne and B. E. L. Long, RCGP, London) and *The Consultation: an Approach to Learning and Teaching* (1984, by D. Pendleton, T. Schofield, P. Tate and P. Havelock, Oxford University Press, Oxford) cover this area well.

You decide that hormone replacement therapy might be appropriate for Mrs Drummond-Brown.

4   *What information and advice would you give her about this treatment?*

This is a straightforward question and clearly demands a degree of factual knowledge about the subject. However, it is much easier to access the knowledge you have and avoid missing anything out if you have a logical approach.

When prescribing any drug it is important to explain to the patient, at a level they can understand, what the drug is intended to do, what side effects may be experienced, whether there are any significant risks involved and how they may be minimized, and how long it will take to act. In addition, they need to know how and when to take the drug and what follow-up is required, if any.

YOU HAVE NOW COMPLETED APPROXIMATELY ONE-HALF OF THE PAPER

Six months later, while staying with her son, Mrs Drummond-Brown is admitted to hospital 30 miles away with a myocardial infarction. Shortly afterwards her son comes to see you. He says that you should not have prescribed hormone replacement therapy 'because it causes thrombosis'.

5   *Outline the points you would wish to cover in your interview with him.*

Once again, a type of question frequently encountered in the MEQ. The management of a patient or relative with a grievance, real or imagined, is something which you should have had plenty of opportunity to explore via video, discussion and role-play both within the practice and on the day-release course. It is important not to react aggressively but to explore the complainant's grievance thoroughly before embarking on an explanation or justification of your own or another doctor's actions. You must also consider confidentiality and any associated ethical problems.

Mrs Drummond-Brown returns to your care. Some months later at follow-up she admits to you that she and her husband have not had sexual intercourse since her heart attack.

6   *What are the possible reasons for this?*

This questions asks you to speculate on the possible underlying causes of this not uncommon sequel to myocardial infarction. If you use your imagination and your previous knowledge of the patient and remember to think in physical, psychological and social terms you should have little difficulty. Remember, though, that sexual problems are rarely entirely unilateral and do not forget to take her husband into account.

She later confides to you that she has noticed a lump in her right breast for several weeks. On examination you find a hard mobile mass 2 cm in diameter below the right nipple and decide this is probably a cancer of the breast. You tell Mrs Drummond-Brown that you wish to refer her immediately to a specialist. Mrs Drummond-Brown says to you: 'If this is a cancer, are there any forms of treatment other than having a breast removed? I couldn't bear that.'

7   *What areas do you wish to explore with her?*

Patient's fears and anxieties about referral to hospital and, in particular, surgical procedures are real and understandable. In addition, mastectomy is rightly seen as a mutilating operation and most intelligent patients are aware that there is considerable debate among doctors as to the appropriate treatment of carcinoma of the breast. Thus, it is important to take into account her own experience and knowledge and any other factors which might colour her attitude towards the disease. What can you do or say to reassure her?

You decide to refer Mrs Drummond-Brown to a specialist.

8   *List the points you would cover in your letter of referral.*

In the same way that you should have developed a systematic approach to history taking, examination, investigation, prescribing and management, so you should have a scheme for writing referral letters. These must include social and demographic details, previous history and allergies, present history, examination findings, investigations performed and current medication. In addition, it is most important to include a note about what the patient has been told and what her fears and expectations are. Most consultants welcome it if the GP makes clear whether the referral is for help with diagnosis or management, a technical procedure or simply for moral support.

Robyn Dowie's book *General Practitioners and Consultants: A study of Outpatient Referrals* (1983, Oxford University Press, Oxford) demonstrates clearly the inadequacy of many referrals and the response to them!

In the event, Mrs Drummond-Brown is treated by simple mastectomy and cytotoxic drugs and after completion of treatment continues to return to the hospital at 3-monthly intervals. You arrange to see her for follow-up as well.

9   *What aspects of her health would you wish to monitor?*

This lady has suffered two major blows to her health and self-esteem over the two years or so covered by this MEQ. The final question often asks you either to review the saga and comment on it, or look forward to future problems which may arise in the patient or the family. Provided that you consider all the parties involved, and range widely over physical, psychological and social factors, you should find it quite easy to gain high marks.

THE ANSWERS TO MEQ TEST 2 APPEAR ON PAGE 95

As you drive into your surgery one morning you are almost in collision with a young man in an old car, who you vaguely recognize as a patient of your partner. His passenger is a patient of yours, Joanna Franklin, a girl of about 17 years, who you know quite well.

A few minutes later you are asked by the receptionist to sign a repeat presciption for phenytoin. Further enquiry reveals that the patient concerned is the driver of the car.

1   *What practical and ethical dilemmas does this situation present you with?*
   How might you resolve them?

Your partner is on holiday, so the young man, whose name is John Fletcher, comes in to see you the next day. Your investigations suggest that he should not be driving.

2   *In what ways might you handle this consultation?*
   What are the pros and cons of each?

A few weeks later Joanna comes to see you herself. She is the only daughter of older, middle-class parents who have considerable expectations of her. She is a sixth-form pupil at the local comprehensive school and is due to take her A levels next year.

She tells you that she is finding it increasingly difficult to keep up with the work. She is constantly tired, irritable and unable to concentrate.

3   *Why might she be presenting in this manner?*
    How would you proceed with the consultation?

It transpires that Joanna is worried because her period is overdue and contraception has been intermittent. You confirm that she is indeed about 8 weeks' pregnant. She breaks down in tears and tells you that she cannot possibly go on with the pregnancy.

4 *What further information do you need to know in order to counsel her effectively? What options does she have?*

YOU HAVE NOW COMPLETED APPROXIMATELY ONE-HALF OF THE PAPER

Eventually Joanna decides to give up her studies, continue with the pregnancy and leave home to live in a flat with her boyfriend. She tells you that her parents are very upset and will not have anything to do with them.

A few days later you receive an abusive letter from her parents. They indicate that it is your fault that Joanna has taken this decision.

5   *How might you respond to this?*
    What are the advantages and disadvantages of each type of response?

Joanna's pregnancy continues uneventfully, but when she comes up to the antenatal clinic at 36 weeks, she tells you that she has had some vaginal discharge for the past few days and feels sore 'down below'.

6   *What are the possible causes of these symptoms?*
   Indicate how you would manage each of them.

Joanna eventually delivers normally at term after a rather long labour. The baby is a boy, who they name Philip. He is breast fed and appears to be making satisfactory progress.

However, when he is about 4 weeks old, Joanna brings him up to see you. She tells you that she is very worried about him because he has been vomiting after feeds ever since she put him on the bottle. You are unable to find any obvious cause for the vomiting and his weight is satisfactory.

7   *What explanations can you suggest for this presentation?*
   What are your management options now?

Philip's feeding problems resolve and he subsequently becomes a rather hyperactive and unruly toddler. Joanna consults you about his behaviour and complains about her tiredness and tension headaches.

As the consultation progresses Philip becomes increasingly unruly and disruptive and chaos treatens to ensue.

8   *In what ways might you cope with the disturbance to the consultation caused by Philip's behaviour?*
What are the advantages and disadvantages of each?

THE ANSWERS TO MEQ TEST 3 APPEAR ON PAGE 105

Late one evening you receive an urgent call about a patient who is new to your list. She is a lady in her late thirties called Pamela Newnham. Her husband tells you that she is 'in a terrible state' and he doesn't know what to do with her.

Further questioning reveals that she is shaking and trembling, finding it difficult to breathe and 'looks awful'. You agree to visit at once. As you drive to her home, you consider the possible diagnoses.

1 (a) List these in order of probability.

(b) How would you approach this diagnostic problem on arrival at the house?

You discover that Mrs Newnham has had several similar attacks in the recent past, but this is by far the worst. She has recently remarried after a divorce and has a mentally handicapped daughter, Mandy (16), and a son, Jake (9), from her first marriage. Her new husband has a teenage son from his previous marriage who is proving to be a considerable problem. You can find no physical abnormality and decide that Mrs Newnham is experiencing an acute panic attack.

2   *What options do you have for managing:*
   (a) The immediate situation.

   (b) The longer-term problems of this patient.

You develop a reasonable relationship with Mrs Newnham and she seems to improve. She tells you that her most pressing problem is the behaviour of her stepson, John (18), who is unemployed and frequently comes home drunk and noisy with his friends. She asks if you would see him and 'give him a good talking to'. He is registered with you.

3 *What problems does this request pose for you and how might you resolve them?*

In the event, you have no opportunity to see John because he leaves home and moves away soon afterwards.

At a subsequent consultation, Mrs Newnham is again upset. Her daughter, Mandy, now attends a training centre for the mentally handicapped and, since it is some distance away, she only comes home at weekends. The specialist who attends the centre has suggested that Mandy should either be started on the Pill or be sterilized, since she is at risk of becoming pregnant.

4   *Why might Mrs Newnham be so upset?*
    What can you do to help her?

YOU HAVE NOW COMPLETED APPROXIMATELY ONE-HALF OF THE PAPER

Mrs Newnham reluctantly accepts that Mandy should take the Pill, although she is still not happy about it. She remains stressed but is managing to cope.

The following winter her son, Jake, who normally keeps well and attends school regularly, develops recurrent colds and coughs, associated with wheezing. You suspect he may be developing asthma.

5   *How would you seek to confirm or refute this diagnosis?*
    If confirmed, what would you say to the parents?

Towards the end of the same winter, Mr Newnham makes one of his rare appearances at the surgery. He is in his late forties and works at a local factory. He smokes 20 cigarettes a day and occasionally has a few beers, although he denies heavy drinking. The only significant previous history is of rectal bleeding from haemorrhoids some years previously, treated by injection.

He complains of feeling unusually tired and of a little 'indigestion' which he has had for the past week.

6   *What are the possible causes for this presentation?*

You are unable to find any abnormality and, after discussion, you arrange to see him again a month later. On this occasion, you find his liver to be enlarged and investigations reveal anaemia and abnormal liver function tests. You arrange a consultation with a consultant physician and Mr Newnham is admitted to hospital urgently.

Metastatic carcinoma is suspected and an ultrasound scan confirms metastatic liver disease. Liver biopsy reveals adenocarcinoma, probably of large bowel origin. Mrs Newnham has been told the diagnosis, but her husband has not.

You are called out at 8 p.m. on a Sunday night 2 days after he has been discharged from hospital. You find him in great distress. He has not been able to pass a motion since leaving hospital and is complaining of abdominal and rectal pain. Anal inspection reveals oedematous and angry-looking haemorrhoids. Rectal examination is impossible to perform.

7   *Enumerate the problems which you face at this point.*
    What immediate management options do you have?

Mr Newnham is admitted to hospital and discharged home again within 48 hours passing normal motions without pain.

8   *What can you do to help the members of this family to cope over the weeks and months ahead?*

THE ANSWERS TO MEQ TEST 4 APPEAR ON PAGE 113

Before your next patient enters you look at her problem card (*see* page 151), created by your recently retired partner, whose patient she has been. She has not seen you before.

When Mrs Smith comes in she complains of generalized weakness for which you can find no cause. In the course of the consultation, you elicit that she is worried because her Merchant Seaman husband seems obsessed with the belief that he might have AIDS. She asks if he has consulted you recently.

1   *What would you wish to cover in the ensuing discussion?*

Assessment of the patient's	*2½%*
Physical condition	
Psychological condition	
Social situation	
Assessment of her husband's	*2½%*
Physical condition	
Psychological condition	
Social situation	
With regard to AIDS	*2½%*
Check patient's ideas, concerns and expectations regarding the condition	
Give accurate information in a form and at a level the patient can understand	
Further management	*3%*
Encourage husband's attendance	
Offer further investigation or referral if indicated	
Arrange follow-up	
Stress confidentiality and maintenance of the doctor/patient relationship	*2%*
Total	*12½%*

Some weeks later Mrs Smith attends complaining of pins and needles in her hands and feet. On full examination you can find no abnormality, and the history together with your previous investigations confirms your impression that this is not an organic disorder.

2   (a) *Speculate about the origins of this patient's symptoms.*

      Physical $2\frac{1}{2}\%$
        Neuropathy, e.g. alcohol, diabetes
        Other neurological, e.g. multiple sclerosis (MS)
        Hyperventilation syndrome

      Psychological $2\frac{1}{2}\%$
        Past history of somatization of anxiety
        Experience of loss, e.g. father's death, husband ? ill
        Anxiety about own health, e.g. fear of AIDS, MS or myocardial infarction

      Social $2\frac{1}{2}\%$
        Probable marital difficulties
        Consequences of husband suffering from AIDS, e.g. stigma, deprivation, death

(b) *How can you help her?*

      Personally $1\frac{1}{2}\%$
        Explanation, sympathy, support
        Counselling

      Involve others   1%
        Community Psychiatric Nurse (CPN), social worker, counsellor
        Marriage guidance or family therapy

      Consider further investigation or referral $2\frac{1}{2}\%$
        Pros and cons of testing for antibodies to HIV
        Further search for organic causes
        Pros and cons of referral

                                                                   Total $12\frac{1}{2}\%$

The consultation ends unsatisfactorily. The following day Mr Smith calls to see you, demanding an explanation of his wife's symptoms. He tells you he has made arrangements for her to see a homoeopathic practitioner.

3   **In what ways might you respond?**
       What are the pros and cons of each?

Agree, accept and explain	3%
Pros: pleases patient, saves time	
Cons: avoids the issue, may breach Mrs Smith's confidentiality	
Disagree, reject and refuse	2½%
Pros: maintains confidentiality	
Cons: may disrupt doctor–patient relationship, may exacerbate the problems	
Explore Mr Smith's anger	2½%
Pros: may resolve problems and uncover anxieties	
Cons: time consuming, may be counterproductive	
Explore family dynamics	2½%
Pros: may throw more light on family, marital, sexual relationships	
Cons: time consuming, may be rejected	
Follow-up	2%
Joint consultation with wife	
Offer of help from other agencies if appropriate	

Total   12½%

Six months later Mrs Smith complains of loss of vision in one eye. She sees your partner, who suspects she has retrobulbar neuritis, and refers her to a neurologist. The diagnosis of multiple sclerosis is confirmed by his clinical examination and supported by sensory, visual and auditory evoked responses. Later Mr and Mrs Smith come to see you to discuss the neurologist's report.

4   *List the areas you would wish to consider with them at this consultation.*

Initial assessment of the couple's	2½%
Understanding of the problem	
Feelings about the problem	
Feelings about the doctor	
Discussion about MS	2%
Cause, effect, prognosis etc.	1%
Management	2%
Orthodox methods	
Alternative approaches	
Implications for the future	2½%
Work, family, pregnancy etc.	
Available help	2½%
Follow-up by GP	
Follow-up by specialist	
Help from primary health care team (PHCT), e.g. nurse	
Help from other agencies, e.g. occupational therapy	
Financial support, allowances etc.	

Total   12½%

Some time later Mrs Smith brings Debbie, now aged 6, because of a vaginal discharge. She (Debbie) has recently started wetting the bed again and is off her food.

5 (a) **List the possible causes of this presentation.**

> *Physical*   3%
> *Urinary tract infection*
> *Vaginitis*
> *Foreign body in vagina*
> *Others, e.g. diabetes, worms*
> *Sexual abuse*

> *Psychological*   2%
> *Marital problems*
> *Mother's condition*
> *Father's absences at sea*

> *Social, e.g. problems at school*

(b) **Outline how you would manage this consultation.**

> *Structure of consultation*   1%
> *Consider involving practice nurse or Health Visitor*
> *Consider relationship with child/mother*   2%
> *Consider whether the time available is sufficient and the*
> *circumstances suitable*

> *Further elaboration of history*

> *Examination*   2%
> *General for evidence of illness*
> *Specific for evidence of abuse*

> *Investigation*
> *Mid-stream specimen of urine (MSU), vaginal swab etc.*

> *Management*   2½%
> *Explanation and advice*
> *Consideration of referral*
> *Follow-up*

Total   12½%

Two days later Debbie's schoolteacher phones you in distress. She tells you that Debbie has implied that her father has interfered with her in some way.

6   *What problems does this pose for a GP?*
       How would you deal with them?

How to confirm accuracy of Debbie's story	2%
How to assess the risks to Debbie and her family	2%
How to maintain confidentiality	1½%
Whether to break confidentiality if required by complying with official guidelines and thus involving social services, police etc.	3%
How to communicate your findings to the family and others concerned	1%
How to manage the situation	1%
Within the practice	1%
By using external resources and procedures	1%

Total   12½%

Mr Smith deserts his family and returns to sea. A few days later, Mrs Smith comes to see you. She implies that you have been responsible, to some extent, for the break-up of her marriage. She asks to see her notes to ensure that there is no information recorded which might prejudice her future doctors against her, as she intends to change.

7   *Discuss the different ways in which you might cope with this request to see her notes and the probable consequences of these.*

Explore the reasons for her request	2%
May cause upset or aggression	
May reveal her fears	
May disclose mental illness	2½%
May help to understand her anger	
May preserve doctor–patient relationship	
Refuse access to notes	2½%
May increase anger	
May finally disrupt doctor–patient relationship	
Probably destroy any hopes of salvaging the situation	
Allow access to notes there and then	3%
May provide reassurance	
May cause further misunderstandings	
Destroys confidentiality of other communications, e.g. hospital letters	
Doctor can provide explanation ? justification	
Allow access to notes at later date	2½%
Gives time to discuss situation with partners,	
Medical Defence Union (MDU) etc.	
Provides an opportunity to exclude sensitive material	
(dishonest unless explained)	
Gives doctor opportunity to educate patient regarding notes	
Total	12½%

After consideration, Mrs Smith remains on your list. At 11 p.m. one Saturday evening you receive a telephone call from an anxious neighbour of the Smith family who has been alerted by Debbie knocking on her door. Apparently Mrs Smith is unconscious from an overdose of an antidepressant you had prescribed. You arrange admission to hospital and appropriate care for Debbie.

The following morning you telephone the hospital and discover that Mrs Smith has died.

8   ***Describe the thoughts and feelings you might have at this time and the ways you could cope with them.***

> *Grief*   1½%
> > *Death of relatively young patient*
> > *Sadness for child*
>
> *Guilt*   2½%
> > *Professional failure to recognize potential suicide*
> > *Provision of antidepressants*
> > *Ineffectiveness of management*
>
> *Anger*   2½%
> > *With patient for 'escaping responsibilities'*
> > *With self for professional failure*
> > *With husband for deserting family*
>
> *Relief because intractable problem has been resolved*
>
> *Anxiety*   2%
> > *For professional reputation*
> > *Possibility of complaint*
> > *Debbie's future*
>
> *Ways of coping*   2½%
> > *Support from colleagues*
> > *Learning from adverse outcomes*
> > *Support from spouse and family*
> > *Providing care for Debbie*
> > *Discussion with Medical Defence Union*   1½%
> > *Appropriate displacement activity, e.g. music, sport*
> > *Inappropriate use of alcohol, drugs etc.*
> > *Rationalization and increased maturity*

Total   12½%

Mrs Drummond-Brown, the 47-year-old wife of a senior company executive, presents at your evening surgery without an appointment and demands to be seen straight away. Her manner is so overbearing that she reduces your receptionist to tears. You see her later that session when she greets you with a smile and complains of hot flushes, night sweats and depression.

1   (a) **What reasons can you suggest for the differing ways in which she has presented to you and to your receptionist?**

> *Problems with practice organization*   2%
> > *Previous difficulties*
> > *Current problems with receptionist*
> > *Social relationship with doctor or family*

> *Problems with patient*
> > *Illness (physical or psychological)*   2½%
> > *Behaviour pattern (innate personality, class, unresolved anger)*

(b) **What, if anything, might you say to her about the earlier episode in reception?**

> *After dealing with presenting problem bring up the problem with her*   1%
> > *Listen to her account in order to understand her feelings*
> > *Provide support to receptionist*   3%
> > *Accept personal responsibility*
> > *Say that you will investigate problem as required*
> > *Explain/apologize as required*
> > *Suggest she might apologize to receptionist*   2½%

                                      Total   11%

You establish that she is depressed and that the hot flushes are not of sufficient severity to interfere with her way of life.

2   *List the past and present social factors which might have predisposed her to depression?*

    Past social factors   3%
      Emotional deprivation
        In childhood
        In marriage
      Premature separation from parent(s)
        Death
        Divorce/marital strife

    Present social factors
      Personal   2%
        Alcohol
        Loneliness/isolation
        Loss of physical attractiveness
      Marital/sexual problems   5%
        With husband
        Extramarital affairs
        Frequent separation
        Husband overworking
        Financial state
        Future prospects
      Family problems   2%
        With children
        With elderly relatives

                                                  Total   12%

Two months later she again comes to your surgery and insists that you prescribe hormone replacement therapy.

3   **What would you want to know before deciding to respond to her request?**

Ideas, concerns and expectations	4%
Severity of symptoms	
Personality factors	
Emotional state	
Sexual problems	
Advice from friends/relatives	
Knowledge of hormone replacement therapy	
Expectations of treatment	
History	1½%
Menstrual pattern	
Symptoms referable to oestrogen deficiency	
Contraindications	3%
Vascular disease	
Breast or genital malignancy	
Smoking/medication	
Diabetes/obesity	
Examination	2½%
BP/weight	
Urine	
Vaginal examination + cervical smear	
Breasts	

Investigation: only if indicated after history and examination

Total   11%

You decide that hormone replacement therapy might be appropriate for Mrs Drummond-Brown.

4 *What information and advice would you give her about this treatment?*

Intended effects of drug   2%
  Replace female hormone lacking
  Relieve symptoms

Possible side effects   2%
  Withdrawal bleeding
  Nausea/breast tenderness/fluid retention

Possible risks   3%
  Thrombosis and embolism (smoking)
  Exacerbation of breast malignancy
  Exacerbation of genital malignancy
  Irregular bleeding (D & C)
  Hypertension

How and when to take tablets   1½%
  Cyclical regimen
  Once daily, limited period

Follow-up   2½%
  Regular, before repeats
  Examination ? annually
  Watch for
    Pain or swelling of legs
    Breast problems
    Irregular bleeding

Total   11%

Six months later, while staying with her son, Mrs Drummond-Brown is admitted to hospital 30 miles away with a myocardial infarction. Shortly afterwards her son comes to see you. He says that you should not have prescribed hormone replacement therapy 'because it causes thrombosis'.

5   **Outline the points you would wish to cover in your interview with him.**

Listen with sympathy and understanding   2½%
   Allow him to give vent to anger
   Enquire about information source
   Explain problem of confidentiality

Discuss myocardial infarction   2%
   Risk factors
   Prognosis

Discuss hormone replacement therapy   2½%
   Risks and benefits
   Contraindications
   Follow-up

Patient autonomy   2½%
   Mature, adult person
   Properly informed
   Properly screened

Follow-up and support   3%
   Convalescence, prognosis
   Future management
   ? Family situation
   Opportunistic health education for son, e.g. stop smoking

                                                            Total   12½%

Mrs Drummond-Brown returns to your care. Some months later, at follow-up she admits to you that she and her husband have not had sexual intercourse since her heart attack.

6   *What are the possible reasons for this?*

    Physical   3%
        Effects of myocardial infarction, e.g. angina, left ventricular failure,
        dyspnoea, palpitations
        Side effects of drug therapy
        Gynaecological problems, e.g. effects of oestrogen deficiency

    Psychological/emotional   3%
        Lack of libido
        Fear of heart attack
        Anxiety/depression
        Poor response to stress/vulnerable

    Social   2½%
        Poor marital relationship
        Extramarital relationship
        Other external factors

    Husband   1%
        Impotence ? cause
        Ageing/illness
        Fear of wife's illness   2½%
        Alcohol problem
        Other external factors, e.g. work, financial

                                                    Total   12%

She later confides to you that she has noticed a lump in her right breast for several weeks. On examination you find a hard mobile mass 2 cm in diameter below the right nipple and decide this is probably a cancer of the breast. You tell Mrs Drummond-Brown that you wish to refer her immediately to a specialist. Mrs Drummond-Brown says to you: 'If this is a cancer are there any forms of treatment other than have a breast removed? I couldn't bear that'.

7   *What areas do you wish to explore with her?*

Patient's fears and anxieties	1%
About mastectomy	
About mutilation/body image	
About sexual difficulties	3%
About prognosis including death	
About effects on family	
About effects on work	
Patient's knowledge and sources of information	2½%
About cancer of the breast	
About surgery	
About alternative treatment	
Present situation	3%
Medical	
Gynaecological	
Psychological	
Marital/sexual	
Reassurance and advice	2½%
Treatment	
Prognosis	
Continuing care and support	
Total	12%

You decide to refer Mrs Drummond-Brown to a specialist.

8   **List the points you would cover in your letter of referral.**

Social/personal
    Name, age, address, tel. no., occupation
    Family situation
	1%

Previous and family history
    Breast cancer
    Obstetric/hormonal
    Myocardial infarction
    Psychiatric
    Allergies
	2½%

Present history and findings on examination
    Duration
    Location of lump
    Associated features
    Evidence of metastases
    Current medication
	2½%

Patient's ideas, concerns and expectations
    Told probable diagnosis
    Fears of mastectomy
    Alternative treatment
    Discussion with GP
	2%

Request to consultant
    Confirm diagnosis
    Discuss treatment available
    Availability of GP
    Willingness to follow-up
	2%

Total   10%

In the event, Mrs Drummond-Brown is treated by simple mastectomy and cytotoxic drugs and, after completion of treatment, continues to return to the hospital at 3-monthly intervals. You arrange to see her for follow-up as well.

9   *What aspects of her health would you wish to monitor?*

    Physical   2½%
       Breast
         Local recurrence
         Distant spread
       Heart
         Progress of angina
         Other problems
       Gynaecological   2½%
         Menopausal symptoms
         Contraception
         Screening
       General
         Problems with therapy
         State of health

    Psychological   2½%
       Attitude to scar/self-image
       Acceptance of prosthesis
       Attitude to sex
       Anxiety and/or depression
       Attitude to disease/prognosis

    Social   1%
       Relationship with husband
       Relationship with family/friends

                                      Total   8½%

MEQ
TEST 3

Answers

As you drive into your surgery one morning you are almost in collision with a young man in an old car, who you vaguely recognize as a patient of your partner. His passenger is a patient of yours, Joanna Franklin, a girl of about 17 years, who you know quite well.

A few minutes later you are asked by the receptionist to sign a repeat prescription for phenytoin. Further enquiry reveals that the patient concerned is the driver for the car.

1 *What practical and ethical dilemmas does this situation present you with? How might you resolve them?*

Practical and ethical dilemmas 3%
   Whether to review notes
   Whether to sign prescription or recall patient
   Whether to say anything to partner
   Whether to say anything to patient
   Whether to inform DVLC, Swansea
   Whether to inform Joanna
   Classic dilemma is balancing responsibility for an individual patient against
   responsibility to society as a whole – confidentiality 1%

Resolution 2½%
   Must check notes to ascertain
     Precise diagnosis
     Degree of control of epilepsy
     Diurnal or nocturnal fits.
     Time elapsed since last attack (most GP records would not be reliable enough)
   If clearly fit to drive, because 2½%
     No epileptic attack for more than 2 years, or
     Only sleep attacks for more than 3 years, and
     Not likely to be a source of danger to the public, then
     Sign repeat prescription, because taking medication is not a bar to driving
   If doubtful or clearly unfit to drive 1½%
     Do not sign repeat prescription
     Patient must be seen urgently
   Prior to consultation, seek advice as required 2%
     From partner, who may wish to see patient personally
     From medical adviser, DVLC, Swansea
     From medical defence organization
     From handbook – Medical Aspects of Fitness to drive

Total 12½%

Your partner is on holiday, so the young man, whose name is John Fletcher, comes in to see you the next day. Your investigations suggest that he should not be driving.

2   **In what ways might you handle this consultation?**
     What are the pros and cons of each?

Write prescription without further ado   1½%
   Pros: *quick and easy*
   Cons: *probably illegal, certainly unethical, could have serious medicolegal*
      consequences

Verbal attack   2%
   Pros: *quick, to the point, may be effective*
   Cons: *may provoke verbal or physical response and will probably disrupt*
      relationship
   Cons: *may leave practice and continue to drive illegally*

Review his condition and lifestyle   3%
   Pros: *explores patient's viewpoint (he may not be aware he is driving illegally)*
   Pros: *maintains good relationship*
   Pros: *more likely to take advice if offered in constructive and sympathetic manner*
   Cons: *time consuming, may not accept advice*

If advice to stop driving and inform DVLC accepted   2%
   Prescribe medication
   Arrange further support and follow-up.
   Pros: *outcome acceptable to all*
   Cons: *limitation of his lifestyle*

If not accepted, or he denies driving, then   4%
   Confront him
   Point out he is driving illegally
   Emphasize the risks he is incurring to himself and others
   Inform him that he is obliged by law to report a 'prescribed disability' to DVLC
   If he remains adamant, inform him that you will be obliged to inform
   DVLC yourself
   Pros: *doctor complying with law*
   Cons: *potential breach of confidentiality*
   Cons: *disruption of doctor–patient relationship, will probably leave practice*

                                                          Total   12½%

A few weeks later Joanna comes to see you herself. She is the only daughter of older, middle-class parents who have considerable expectations of her. She is a sixth-form pupil at the local comprehensive school and is due to take her A levels next year.

She tells you that she is finding it increasingly difficult to keep up with the work. She is constantly tired, irritable and unable to concentrate.

3   *Why might she be presenting in this manner?*
     How would you proceed with the consultation?

Physical (unlikely), e.g. anaemia, infection, pregnancy	1%

Psychological (more likely)
    Anxiety state
    Depression
    Addiction
    Adolescent identity crisis
    Early psychosis
	2%

Social (quite likely)
    Academic difficulties
    Difficulties with parents/family
    Difficulties with boyfriend
	2%

Explore her problems (patient-centred)
    Allow her to talk
    Identify her ideas, concerns and expectations
	2%

Clarify history (doctor-centred)
    Physical
    Psychological
    Social
	2%

Physical examination and investigation *As indicated by history*	1%
Agree on major problems/difficulties	
Explore management options	
Reassure, support	2½%
Stress confidentiality	
Arrange follow-up	

Total 12½%

It transpires that Joanna is worried because her period is overdue and contraception has been intermittent. You confirm that she is indeed about 8 weeks' pregnant. She breaks down in tears and tells you that she cannot possibly go on with the pregnancy.

4   *What further information do you need to know in order to counsel her effectively? What options does she have?*

Her boyfriend	2%
Serious or casual	
Does he know?	
What is his attitude to the pregnancy?	
Will he support her?	
Her parents	2%
Do they know or suspect?	
Could she confide in them?	
What are their general attitudes?	
Herself	2½%
Attitude to pregnancy	
Attitude to abortion	
Any religious convictions?	
Financial position	
Options	
Continue with the pregnancy, and keep the baby	2%
Stay at home or	
Seek help via charity/local services or	
Live with/marry boyfriend	
Continue with the pregnancy and have baby adopted	1%
Seek a termination of pregnancy	2%
NHS	
Clinic	
Privately	
Abandon education	
Continue education at school or elsewhere	1%
Total	12½%

Eventually Joanna decides to give up her studies, continue with the pregnancy, and leave home to live in a flat with her boyfriend. She tells you that her parents are very upset and will not have anything to do with them.

A few days later you receive an abusive letter from her parents. They indicate that it is your fault that Joanna has taken this decision.

5   *How might you respond to this?*
       What are the advantages and disadvantages of each type of response?

Respond positively	2½%
By phone or letter	
By personal visit	
Arrange a meeting	
Discuss with partners ± PHCT	
Advantages	2%
Allows parents to air feelings	
May help parents' guilt	
May improve doctor–patient communication	
May improve family relationships	
May avoid official complaint	
May avoid physical violence	
May avoid removal from list	
Disadvantages	2%
May provoke confrontation	
May disrupt doctor–patient relationship irreversibly	
May further damage family relationships	
Respond negatively	2%
Ignore letter	
React aggressively by phone or letter	
Remove from list	
Consult a medical defence organization (MDU)	
Consult legal adviser	
Communicate with Joanna ? confidentiality	
Advantages	2%
May relieve doctor's feelings	
May terminate unsatisfactory relationship	
May protect doctor's interests	
Disadvantages	2%
May provoke official complaint	
Will disrupt relationship	
May miss opportunity of improving family relationships	

Total   12½%

Joanna's pregnancy continues uneventfully, but when she comes up to the antenatal clinic at 36 weeks, she tells you that she has had some vaginal discharge for the past few days and feels sore 'down below'.

6   *What are the possible causes of these symptoms?*
       Indicate how you would manage each of them.

Common infections	3%
Candida *sp.*	
Investigation, antifungal therapy	
Trichomonas *sp.*	
Investigation, metronidazole	

Less common, but important infections	3%
Gonorrhoea	
Investigation/referral, specific treatment before delivery	
Non-specific urethritis	
Invesigation/referral, specific treatment	
Herpes gestationis	
Investigation/referral ? need for lower segment caesarean section (LSCS)	

No obvious physical cause   3%
   Physiological discharge ⎫
   Trauma from intercourse ⎬ *explanation*
   Sexual problem   *and*
   Anxiety re pregnancy ⎬ *follow-up*
   Anxiety re labour ⎭

Other causes	2½%
Urinary tract infection	
Investigation, specific treatment	
Glycosuria/diabetes	
Investigation, specific treatment	
Local problems	
Chemical irritation – advice	
Bartholin's abscess – referral	
Skin disorder – specific treatment	

Obstetric	1%
Leaking liquor	
Investigation/referral	

Total   12½%

Joanna eventually delivers normally at term after a rather long labour. The baby is a boy, who they name Philip. He is breast fed and appears to be making satisfactory progress.

However, when he is about 4 weeks old, Joanna brings him up to see you. She tells you that she is very worried about him because he has been vomiting after feeds ever since she put him on the bottle. You are unable to find any obvious cause for the vomiting and his weight is satisfactory.

7   *What explanations can you suggest for this presentation?*
    What are your management options now?

Physical in baby	2%
Feeding problem	
Hiatus hernia	
Pyloric stenosis	
General illness	
Allergy to cows' milk	
Psychological in mother	2%
Puerperal depression	
Maternal anxiety	
Ignorance of normality	
Social in family/community	2%
Marital problems	
Problems with grandparents	
Isolation	
Management options	
Baby	2½%
Further history	
Further examination	
Watch feeding	
Treat intercurrent illness	
Refer	
Admit	
Mother	2%
Assess psychological state	
Observe	
Treat	
Refer	
Family	2%
Counselling	
Involvement of family/friends	
Involvement of health visitor	
Observe	
Follow-up	

Total   12½%

Philip's feeding problems resolve and he subsequently becomes a rather hyperative and unruly toddler. Joanna consults you about his behaviour and complains about her tiredness and tension headaches.

As the consultation progresses Philip becomes increasingly unruly and disruptive and chaos threatens to ensue.

8   *In what ways might you cope with the disturbance to the consultation caused by Philip's behaviour?*
     What are the advantages and disadvantages of each?

    Distract Philip, e.g. sweets, toys etc.   2%
        Advantages – observe responses and play
        Disadvantages – only temporary

    Ask nurse or receptionist to take him   2%
        Advantages – allows concentration on Joanna
        Disadvantages
            Philip will feel excluded
            May increase upset
            No opportunity to observe relationship

    Ignore him   2%
        Advantages – probably nil
        Disadvantages
            Doctor distracted
            Mother distracted
            Relationship deteriorates
            Damage to surgery

    Control Philip personally   2%
        Advantages – may be educational for mother and child
        Disadvantages – may aggravate problem

    Observe mother–child relationship and comment upon it   2½%
        Advantages
            May help understand problem
            May help to give specific useful advice
        Disadvantages – ignores Joanna's presenting problems

    Terminate the consultation, and arrange to see Joanna alone   2%
        Advantages – allows uninterrupted consultation
        Disadvantages
            May not come
            May feel rejected
            Time-consuming

Total   12½%

Late one evening you receive an urgent call about a patient who is new to your list. She is a lady in her late thirties called Pamela Newnham. Her husband tells you that she is 'in a terrible state' and he doesn't know what to do with her.

Further questioning reveals that she is shaking and trembling, finding it difficult to breathe and 'looks awful'. You agree to visit at once. As you drive to her home, you consider the possible diagnoses.

1 (a) List these in order of probability.

Psychological (most likely)   3%
  Panic attack
  Alcohol or drug withdrawal
  Other reasonable suggestions

Physical (less likely)   2%
  Pneumothorax
  Pulmonary embolus
  Asthma
  Chest infection
  Cardiac arrhythmia
  Other reasonable suggestions

(b) *How would you approach this diagnostic problem on arrival at the house?*

Initial assessment   2%
  'Atmosphere' of home
    Tense, hostile, chaotic etc.
  Response to doctor from patient and family

Conduct of consultation   2%
  Calm and confident
  Sit down next to patient for reassurance and support

History   2%
  Previous attacks
  Onset of present attack
  Progress of present attack
  Any medication?
  Psychosocial factors

Examination/investigation (as indicated by history, but must include)   2%
  General appearance (respiratory distress, cyanosis, pallor etc.)
  Cardiovascular system
  Respiratory system
  Other as indicated
  Peak flow, ECG etc. if indicated

                                                    Total   13%

You discover that Mrs Newnham has had several similar attacks in the recent past, but this is by far the worst. She has recently remarried after a divorce and has a mentally handicapped daughter, Mandy (16), and a son, Jake (9), from her first marriage. Her new husband has a teenage son from his previous marriage who is proving to be a considerable problem. You can find no physical abnormality and decide that Mrs Newnham is experiencing an acute panic attack.

2   *What options do you have for managing:*

   (a) *The immediate situation.*

   Patient and family centred (listen, explain, calm, reassure)

   Doctor centred (confront, be firm, reprove)   4%

   Help her control overbreathing (explanation, re breathe from bag)

   Administer tranquillizer, e.g. benzodiazepine or alternative

   May consider urgent psychiatric referral or admission if indicated

   (b) *The longer-term problems of this patient.*

   Personal follow-up   1%
      In surgery or at home to explore problems further   1%
      To reduce anxiety and enable her to gain control of panic attacks   3%
         By counselling techniques including transactional analysis (TA)
         By medication (risk of dependence)
         By behavioural techniques
         By hypnosis
         By family therapy

   Referral   2%
      Within PHCT, e.g. community psychiatric nurse, psychologist
      To group therapy
      To psychiatrist (domiciliary visit, outpatients or admission)

   Removal from list and leave problem to another doctor   1%
                                                                                          _____
                                                                             Total   12%
                                                                                          _____

You develop a reasonable relationship with Mrs Newnham and she seems to improve. She tells you that her most pressing problem is the behaviour of her stepson, John (18), who is unemployed and frequently comes home drunk and noisy with his friends. She asks if you would see him and 'give him a good talking to'. He is registered with you.

3   *What problems does this request pose for you and how might you resolve them?*

    Doctor–patient relationship   2%
      Need to support Mrs Newnham
      Seen to be intervening positively
      May help family situation
      Need to explore husband's viewpoint

    Ethical   2%
      Does John want advice?
      Will he accept advice?
      Autonomous adult
      Confidentiality

    Practical   2%
      How to contact him?
        Via mother (may provoke hostility)
        Via telephone or letter
        Via 'casual' visit
      Wait until he next comes to surgery

    If contact is achieved   2%
      How to raise topic?
      Drinking, history and effects
      His acceptance of the problem
      His willingness to comply

    Involvement of outside agencies   2%
      Community psychiatric nurse, psychologist, social worker, psychiatrist
      Alcoholics Anonymous

    Resolution   3%
      Assure Mrs Newnham of your support
      Explain ethical and practical problems
      Try to arrange meeting with John
      If successful, manage as appropriate
      If not, record on notes and await opportunity

                                                    Total   13%

In the event, you have no opportunity to see John because he leaves home and moves away soon afterwards.

At a subsequent consultation, Mrs Newnham is again upset. Her daughter, Mandy, now attends a training centre for the mentally handicapped and, since it is some distance away, she only comes home at weekends. The specialist who attends the centre has suggested that Mandy should either be started on the Pill or be sterilized, since she is at risk of becoming pregnant.

4   *Why might Mrs Newnham be so upset?*
       What can you do to help her?

Why upset?	6%
Awareness of Mandy's vulnerability	
Awareness of Mandy's sexuality	
Reminder of own sexuality/jealousy	
Awareness of recent publicity/stigma	
Anger at 'inadequate supervision'	
Guilt about allowing other people to care for daughter	
Religious/moral objections	
Risk of side effects of Pill	
Risk of sexually transmitted diseases, AIDS	
Risk of sterilization operation	
Possible legal complications	
What might family/friends, neighbours say?	
How to help	3%
Express sympathy and support	
Stress confidentiality	
Use counselling techniques to	
Help her air her thoughts and feelings	
Help her understand the problem	
Help her come to terms with Mandy's maturity	
Examine alternative options	3%
Offer to communicate with doctor/staff	
Offer to see Mandy	
Refuse permission for contraception/sterilization	
Withdraw Mandy from training centre	
? any alternatives	

Total   12%

Mrs Newnham reluctantly accepts that Mandy should take the Pill, although she is still not happy about it. She remains stressed but is managing to cope.

The following winter her son, Jake, who normally keeps well and attends school regularly, develops recurrent colds and coughs, associated with wheezing. You suspect he may be developing asthma.

5   *How would you seek to confirm or refute this diagnosis?*
      If confirmed, what would you say to the parents?

Confirmation	
History	2%
Any family history of asthma?	
Any history of atopy	
Details of previous episodes	
Precipitating factors? e.g. exercise, cold air, upper respiratory tract infection	
Examination	2%
Observation during attack	
Auscultation of chest	
Investigation/treatment/referral	2%
Demonstration of reversible airways obstruction by peak-flow meter,	
after use of inhaler or nebulizer	
What to say to parents	
Explore their ideas, concerns and expectations	3%
What do they think, fear?	
Have they considered asthma?	
What does 'asthma' mean to them?	
Explanation	3%
About asthma (honest, open)	
Nature, prognosis, significance	
Avoidance of precipitating factors	
Stress good treatment available	
Explain how they can help	
Provide written material, e.g. leaflet	
Stress importance of helping Jake live a normal life.	

Total   12%

Towards the end of the same winter, Mr Newnham makes one of his rare appearances at the surgery. He is in his late forties and works at a local factory. He smokes 20 cigarettes a day and occasionally has a few beers, although he denies heavy drinking. The only significant previous history is of rectal bleeding from haemorrhoids some years previously, treated by injection.

He complains of feeling unusually tired and of a little 'indigestion' which he has had for the past week.

6   ***What are the possible causes for this presentation?***

Physical (quite likely, in view of his age and infrequent attendance)   3%
  Anaemia ? secondary to peptic ulcer
  Malignancy, e.g. stomach, lung, bowel
  Endocrine disorder
  Infection
  Other reasonable suggestions

Psychological (unlikely, in view of previous history)   3%
  Endogenous depression
  Anxiety
  Alcohol or drug abuse
  Sexual problems, e.g. impotence
  Other reasonable suggestions

Social (quite likely, in view of his family problems)   4%
  Unresolved problems with first wife, divorce etc.
  Unresolved problems with son (alcohol)
  Financial problems
  Employment problems
  Problems with stepson (asthma)
  Problems with stepdaughter (handicapped)
  Problems with elderly parents – bereavement
  Other reasonable suggestions

Marital (quite likely)   3%
  Conflict with wife
    Over stepchildren
    Personal relationship
    Over sex (frigidity etc.)
  Extramarital affairs
  Wife exhausted, ill, depressed
  Other reasonable suggestions

Total   13%

You are unable to find any abnormality and, after discussion, you arrange to see him again a month later. On this occasion, you find his liver to be enlarged and investigations reveal anaemia and abnormal liver function tests. You arrange a consultation with a consultant physician and Mr Newnham is admitted to hospital urgently.

Metastatic carcinoma is suspected and an ultrasound scan confirms metastatic liver disease. Liver biopsy reveals adenocarcinoma, probably of large bowel origin. Mrs Newnham has been told the diagnosis, but her husband has not.

You are called out at 8 p.m. on a Sunday night 2 days after he has been discharged from hospital. You find him in great distress. He has not been able to pass a motion since leaving hospital and is complaining of abdominal and rectal pain. Anal inspection reveals oedematous and angry-looking haemorrhoids. Rectal examination is impossible to perform.

7 *Enumerate the problems which you face at this point.*
What immediate management options do you have?

Practical problems	*3%*
How to resolve the patient's pain and discomfort?	
Does he need readmission to hospital?	
If so, will he accept readmission	
Emotional problems	
Mr Newnham is ill, in pain and unaware of his diagnosis	*1%*
Mrs Newnham is likely to be anxious, upset and 'keeping a secret'	*1%*
The doctor may be	
Guilty because of the delay in diagnosis ?one month ?several years	*1%*
Upset because of the implications of the diagnosis	*1%*
Angry with the hospital for not informing him/her of discharge	*1%*
Angry with the hospital for sharing the diagnosis with the wife alone	*1%*
Management options	*4%*
Treat at home	
Ice-pack, local cream or suppository sedation	
Domiciliary consultation	
With consultant surgeon	
Urgent readmission	
For general anaesthetic, anal dilatation, bowel evacuation	

Total 13%

Mr Newnham is admitted to hospital and discharged home again within 48 hours passing normal motions without pain.

8   *What can you do to help the members of this family to cope over the weeks and months ahead?*

General   4%
   Offer continuing care, sympathy, support and availability
   Involve PHCT, especially community nurses
   Consider involving local hospice team if appropriate
   Promote an atmosphere of shared acceptance, understanding and care

Specific
   Mr Newnham   3%
      Provide effective terminal care
      Relief of pain and discomfort
      Referral as appropriate
      Share diagnosis and prognosis with him when he is ready
      Accept his inevitable anger, frustration and sense of loss
   Mrs Newnham   3%
      Discuss diagnosis with her and encourage 'openness'
      Prepare her for bereavement
      Be aware if she is finding the strain unbearable and take appropriate action
   Children   2%
      Be aware that Mandy may have difficulty in appreciating situation –
      advise training centre
      Be aware that Jake may have unresolved problems re his stepfather
      Be aware that John, his own son, may reappear to seek reconciliation if he
      knows his father is dying

                                                                            Total   12%

Critical reading question paper

The MRCGP examination is currently (Autumn 1990) undergoing a major review. It has been agreed by College Council that a new question paper, the *Critical Reading* paper, will replace the *Practice Topic Question* paper in October 1990.

The examination has, since its inception in 1968, contained a Practice Topic Question (formerly the Traditional Essay Question) which has presented the candidate with the opportunity to organise and display knowledge, and indicate skills and attitudes, on any topic of relevance to general practice. The questions asked in the past were usually related to a broad clinical issue, an aspect of human development or behaviour, and an issue in the general area of practice management.

Limitations of the Practice Topic Question

Whilst, in the past, essays have been an acceptable method of assessment, it has become increasingly recognised that they are difficult to mark reliably, even with well-planned marking schedules. Also, because such a small number of areas and attributes are sampled in any one examination paper, the essay format is a less reliable guide to the general ability of the candidate than many other available methods. The development work being undertaken has confirmed that the *Practice Topic Question* paper has the same failings as all other medical essay papers.

Critical Reading paper

The Examination Board of the Royal College of General Practitioners wants all candidates to display their full potential and to have an examination which reliably measures ability. To this end the examination must be both fair to the candidate, relevant to everyday practice, and appropriate to the needs of general practice as a whole. The Critical Reading paper will assess the candidate's ability to understand, summarize and critically evaluate one or more published papers and written material encountered in general practice. The ability to apply what has been read will also be tested.

Candidates will also be expected to be familiar with, and demonstrate the ability to evaluate, significant published literature on current topics in general practice and to recognise the implications of such literature to their work as a doctor.

The examination is oriented towards general practice in Britain and candidates are advised to concentrate their reading on the reputable books and journals commonly available to British general practitioners. Major publications from overseas which have influenced British general practice should also be considered (Dwyer, 1990).

The paper will be of two hours' duration although an additional 15 minutes will be allowed for candidates to read the presented material. The paper will normally contain three questions, each carrying equal marks. The subject matter will cover the areas of 'health and disease', 'medicine and society' and 'practice management'. Candidates are advised to present their answers in expanded note form unless otherwise instructed.

Question 1

In question 1, candidates will be presented with a published paper from an established general medical journal relevant to British general practice and will be tested on their ability to recognise the main issues raised, comment where appropriate on the design of the study and discuss the implications and practical application of the results to general practice.

Example

Brice, F. C. *et al.* (1990) General Practitioner obstetrics in Bradford. *British Medical Journal*, **300**, 725–727 (Please note that the published paper used in question 1 will be presented without the abstract)

Question 1

(a) List the main points made in this paper.
(b) Comment briefly on the design of the study and the presentation of the results (method and results section of the paper).
(c) If the conclusions of this paper were supported by further research, list the implications to you as a general practitioner.

Question 2

In question 2, candidates will be examined on their familiarity with published literature in areas of current interest in general practice. Marks will be given for demonstrating factual knowledge and mentioning references, but the majority of marks will be awarded to those who show they have read and understood relevant literature on the subject.

Example

Question 2

Summarize, with appropriate evidence, current views on the following:

(a) the use of thrombolytics in the acute management of myocardial infarcts;
(b) factors influencing patient's choice of general practitioner;
(c) the incidence of myalgic encephalomyelitis.

Question 3

In question 3 candidates will be presented with written material commonly encountered in general practice and asked to analyse and respond to it. For example, this may take the form of a letter, a practice protocol, a practice report, a practice audit or advertising material. Candidates will be expected to demonstrate the ability to analyse the practical implications of the presented material in their work as general practitioners.

Example

Question 3

Dear David

Deborah . . . . dob 26/6/75

This patient came to see me today without a letter. She is only 15 years old and is pregnant and has had four sexual partners in her short life. She attended the Family Planning Clinic and saw a lady doctor with glasses but was refused contraception before she became pregnant. I think this is a *terrible* mistake and ought not to happen nowadays. She is eight weeks' pregnant. I am prepared to do a termination of pregnancy on her but we have the problem that she is under sixteen and we need someone to sign the consent form. Could you think about this one because she refuses absolutely to tell her mother and father. She says that if she tells her parents that she is pregnant, she will be thrown out of the house.

Yours sincerely

Mr   FRCOG
Consultant Gynaecologist/Obstetrician

PS   Perhaps you could tell the Family Planning doctor of my comments.

(a) **What are the issues raised by the letter from the consultant gynaecologist?**
(b) **What are your options for management?**
(c) **Give reasons for your favoured approach.**

Reference

Dwyer, D. (1990) The Critical Reading Question paper – a new paper in the MRCGP examination. *Postgraduate Education in General Practice*, **1**, 117–118.

General Reading

Gore, S. M. and Altman, D. G. (1982) *Statistics in practice*, pp. 1–24. British Medical Association, London.
Gore, S. M. and Altman, D. G. (1990) *Guidelines on writing papers*, pp. 38–40. British Medical Association, London.
Jewell, D. (1988) Reading Scientific articles or how to cope with the overload. *Practitioner*, **232**, 720–725.
Sackett, D. L., Hayes, R. B. and Tugwell, P. (1985) *Clinical epidemiology: a basic science for clinical medicine*. Little, Brown & Co, Boston.
Swinton, T. D. V. (1981) *Statistics at square one: articles published in the British Medical Journal*. 3rd edition. British Medical Association, London.

E Gambrill
A Moulds
J Fry
D Brooks

September 1990

Practice Topic Question or PTQ

A new name has not altered the Traditional Essay Question in any essential way. The paper assesses the candidate's ability to develop an argument or statement logically and in writing. Knowledge has to be organized and expressed critically, clearly and succinctly. At least one question in each paper is likely to test attitudes towards innovative, radical or even controversial developments in general practice.

The time available is 2 hours and candidates have to answer three questions one of which may well be divided into two or three parts. Although there is no choice the time allowed is just about adequate. Remember to restrain any tendency to 'allow the pen to flow'. Word economy rather than literary 'largesse' is an important concept to grasp.

Attempts are made 'to balance' the paper in that questions are selected from all five areas of general practice:

Area one   Clinical practice – health and disease.

Area two   Clinical practice – human development.

Area three   Human behaviour.

Area four   Medicine and society.

Area five   The practice.

Any question in areas one and two would certainly expect a 'general practitioner approach' concentrating on assessment and management rather than on pathophysiology. The paper would be balanced by including questions on 'human behaviour' or 'medicine and society' or 'the practice'.

Examiners are people who work at and are interested in the developing frontiers of general practice. The questions and topics that are exercising their minds, therefore, will be those that the discipline is currently addressing. To an extent therefore questions can be predicted by tuning in through reading, understanding, arguing and developing leading articles and position statements which appear in the College journal, other journals such as *Update* and to a lesser extent the *British Medical Journal*. A day-release group is an excellent forum for this sort of activity.

A candidate who relies on reading without opening his or her mind to the views of others in this way is more likely to fail.

Marking

Each question is marked by two examiners independently using cribs or marking grids which allocate approximately 70 per cent of the marks to content. Up to 30 per cent of the marks are discretionary and are awarded for presentation, coherence of argument presented, balance and so on.

The marking schedules we have given for the mock tests are not the same as those used by examiners which are much more concise and are really a point-by-point check list. We are trying to inform as well as test so we have given model answers rather than marking grids as we felt this would be more helpful. Please remember that in the examination, shorter, tighter answers can also score high marks.

Technique

Roughly equal time (40 minutes) should be allotted for each question. It is far harder to gain the last 30–40 per cent of marks for a question than it is to attain the first 30–40 per cent.

Before starting to write, read the question carefully, then spend 5–10 minutes collecting your thoughts; make brief notes of areas or points to cover; jot down your main headings. Then build the notes into the essay itself, remembering that a well constructed, legible essay makes a good impact on the examiner and will attract discretionary marks.

Repetition and lengthy wordiness distract the examiner and make it difficult for him or her to find the nuggets among the dross. Do not pad your answers out. When you have nothing else to say, stop.

A good essay will be based on:

Logical sequence – beginning with an introduction and ending with a conclusion.
Relevant content – directly and appropriately answering the question posed.
Clear and succinct presentation – written legibly in paragraphs with short sentences. Spaced attractively with liberal use of headings and having important points or headings underlined.

Examples of excellent answers from the exam itself can be found in the *Journal of the RCGP* of November 1983 (Volume 33, Number 256) on pp. 735–7.

How to 'diverge'

Most of us tend to think convergently in that we focus down (like a long focus lens) onto a theme that interests us, forgetting in the process large chunks of relevant material at the periphery of our mental vision. We need a structure or a template that allows us to 'open up' ensuring that nothing that could be relevant is neglected.

Question

Discuss factors which influence prescribing rates.

Technique

After an appropriate introduction which says what the rates are and how they vary, why not apply the five areas of general practice as a 'template'? This allows us to jot down topics that spring to mind in each area.

1 Area one
   - Nature of the illness or problem
   - The availability of an effective pharmacological remedy
2 Area two
   - The effect of childhood and old age on our 'prescribing reflex'
   - Different patient expectations at different stages of development
3 Area three
   - Patient ideas, concerns and expections
   - Doctor's interpersonal skills and ability to demonstrate alternative problem-solving strategies
4 Area four
   Patient's and society's attitudes towards taking drugs:
   - Effect of the media
   - Cost of prescribing
        to society
        to the individual
   - Social class differences
5 Area five
   - Age of partners and length of time in practice
   - Accessibility and availability of partners
   - Length of consultation available to patients
   - Quality of reception staff – how easy is it to make an appointment
   - Are prescriptions left for patient to pick up?

Summary

Pros and cons of a high prescription rate.
Some kind of conclusion.

Question

Discuss your management of a young woman of 16 who presents with 'cystitis'.

Technique

After an introduction which explains what 'cystitis' means and discusses its frequency in the community, why not apply Pendleton and Schofield's* seven consultation tasks in order to produce a skeleton answer?

Task 1 To define the reasons for the patient's attendance in physical, psychological and social terms:
- Nature and history of problems
- Aetiology
- Patient's ideas, concerns and expectations (what has she read?)
- Effects of problems (this is often neglected)

Task 2 To consider other problems
- Continuing problems
- At risk factors (contraception if cystitis follows sexual intercourse)

Task 3 To choose an appropriate action for each problem

Task 4 To achieve a shared understanding of the problems with the patient

Task 5 To involve the patient in management and encourage her to accept appropriate responsibility (e.g. dip-slide to take home if chronic problem, self-care with fluids and analgesics)

Task 6 To use time and resources appropriately:
- In the consultation
- Long-term

Task 7 To establish and maintain a relationship with the patient which helps to achieve the other tasks

An alternative approach could be to use a management acronym, e.g. RAPRIOP†:

R Reassurance – no kidney disease; serious troublesome problem unlikely in the future.
A Advice   – fluids, precipitating causes, e.g. sexual intercourse.
P Prescription – 3 days of trimethoprim or self-care if symptoms mild.
R Referral   – unlikely to be necessary.
I Investigation – probably not necessary.
O Observation   – see if problem recurs.
P Prevention   – may be needed if chronic problem develops.

---

* Schofield, T. (1983) The application of the Study of Communication Skills to Training for General Practice. In *Doctor–Patient Communication,* edited by D. Pendleton and J. Hasler, p. 259.
† Fraser, R. (1988) *Clinical Method – A General Practice Approach.* Butterworths, London.

Question

How would you conduct a consultation with a child of six who has an uncomplicated respiratory tract infection?

Technique

A quite sophisticated approach to the problem of generating ideas in a PTQ is by using a matrix and thinking in two dimensions. RAPRIOP is made even more useful by setting it against the five areas of general practice (*see* the table). The boxes can be filled with ideas which spring to mind. Some boxes may be easy to fill, others more difficult. If we produce too many ideas we can always introduce concepts such as 'must do', 'should do' and 'could do' in order to organize priorities. In this way we are thinking in three dimensions (distinction candidates please note)!

Table RAPRIOP against the five areas of general practice – a management matrix for a child of six with an uncomplicated upper respiratory tract infection

	I Clinical medicine	II Human development	III Human behaviour	IV Society and medicine	V The practice
Reassurance	Explain natural history		Mother's concerns and hidden fears	Effects on the family and society	Easy appointments
Advice	Predict the course of the illness	Discuss prevalence at this stage			Using the practice—practice leaflets
Prescription	Simple antipyretic analgesia	Remember asprin and Reye's syndrome	Mother's expectations	Is my script too expensive?	Repeat prescriptions?
Referral			Is Mother confident in my management?		The team?
Investigation				Avoid unnecessary investigation	Practice facilities
Observation	Ask Mother to return *if* predicted course does not occur		Do I need to suggest routine follow-up?		
Prevention	Could this be asthma? Is this child at risk?		Allowing Mother to manage helps her to learn to cope	Need to stay off school?	Leaflets on self-care

Remember

There is no such thing as the perfect template or the perfect matrix. Devising your own and applying them to Practice Topic Questions (either by yourself or in small groups) is an excellent way of preparing for this section of the examination.

Time allowed — 2 hours
All three questions must be answered

Q1 *You have been asked to join a small working party which includes a general practitioner, an obstetrician, a paediatrician and a community midwife. Your brief is to help to develop a protocol for the delivery of antenatal care in your health service district. Outline the content of a discussion paper which you intend to present to the group which outlines the aspects of care you consider to be important and changes that are needed in order to implement them.*

Q2 *A 22-year-old man presents with a 10-day history of 'indigestion' which has been eased to an extent by antacids. Discuss in detail your management plans and the principles which underline them.*

Q3 *Write short notes on:*
A   Hysterectomy.
B   Migraine.

THE ANSWERS TO PTQ TEST 1 BEGIN ON PAGE 131

Time allowed — 2 hours
All three questions must be answered

Q1 'The Medical Profession has become a major threat to health'.
                                                    Ivan Illich, 1977.
    Discuss your reaction to this statement with special reference to the role of the general
    practitioner.

Q2 Discuss in detail the childhood immunization programme, including the contraindica-
    tions to the various vaccines.
        In practice, how would you try to achieve the highest uptake rates possible?

Q3 A 70-year-old man presents with a 3-month history of hesitancy, nocturia, slowness of
    the urine stream and terminal dribbling.
        Discuss in detail how you would care for this patient indicating the likely diagnosis.

THE ANSWERS TO PTQ TEST 2 BEGIN ON PAGE 139

PTQ
TEST 3

Time allowed — 2 hours
All three questions must be answered

Q1 *Discuss the ways in which the GP, the district nurse and the health visitor might cooperate in the delivery of primary health care. Indicate your preferences giving reasons for your choice.*

Q2 *Discuss the ways in which the practice might improve its performance in caring for patients who drink alcohol.*

Q3 *Write short notes on:*
A   Vertigo.
B   Frozen shoulder.

THE ANSWERS TO PTQ TEST 3 BEGIN ON PAGE 147

Time allowed — 2 hours
All three questions must be answered

Q1 Discuss the value of screening for hypertension in general practice. How should case findings be conducted and patients then managed?

Q2 Write short notes on:
A Bedwetting.
B Patient participation groups.

Q3 What is terminal care? Discuss the role of the general practitioner.
How should you respond if a patient you are treating asks about euthanasia?

THE ANSWERS TO PTQ TEST 4 BEGIN ON PAGE 155

Q1 *You have been asked to join a small working party which includes a general practitioner, an obstetrician, a paediatrician and a community midwife. Your brief is to help to develop a protocol for the delivery of antenatal care in your health service district. Outline the content of a discussion paper which you intend to present to the group which outlines the aspects of care you consider to be important and changes that are needed in order to implement them.*

A1 **1. Preamble**

Currently the delivery of antenatal care within most NHS districts is uneconomic, ineffective and probably suboptimally effective. This is because of a dual system of care between hospital and general practice and even a triple system if (as should be the case) the community midwife is included. There is much consumer dissatisfaction.

The following document is a discussion paper which is intended to support the following aims:

- To deliver antenatal care very largely within general practice to all women 'normal' on booking and who remain normal throughout their antenatal care.
- To identify all women at risk who would benefit from an initial consultant opinion and/or an opinion during pregnancy.
- To offer helpful advice on antenatal care in hospital based on a GP viewpoint.
- To reduce attendances to a minimum consistent with the above aims and the establishment of a relationship of trust which will allay maternal anxiety and identify patient ideas, expectations and causes for concern.

10 marks

2. Changes needed

The delivery of antenatal care would be cheaper, more attentive to women's own ideas and more effective if there was:

- A shift away from impersonal and overcrowded antenatal care in hospital outpatient clinics to continuing and personal community care in the GP's surgery.
- A shift away from dubiously 'scientific' care dictated by professionals to care determined by women's own ideas.

5 marks

3. A general practitioner service — priorities

- Early booking allows advice on health matters such as smoking, alcohol and drugs. Early confirmation of pregnancy allows accurate determination of the period of gestation.
- Once pregnancy is confirmed there is a need to allow all women to discuss the pattern of antenatal care which is most suitable and alternatives with regard to place of delivery. This will involve GP, community midwife and possibly the health visitor in all cases.

    The first visit after confirmation should allow a woman to discuss all these things and give her an opportunity to meet all team members involved in care.
- Agreement between the professions locally may allow the practice team to carry out the initial assessment in most cases referring only women in certain categories. In other places the accepted practice may be for all women to be referred to a consultant. Guidelines must be clear to all and allow as much care as possible in the community.

10 marks

4. The initial assessment

- Need for locally agreed checklists during the initial assessment covering important items such as age, parity, height, weight, medical, surgical and obstetric history, alcohol, smoking and diet.
- Women may be considered at high risk in pregnancy and labour due to obstetric causes, e.g. history of low-birth-weight infant, or medical causes, e.g. diabetes. Such women need specialist care during pregnancy and labour.
- Women may be considered a high risk in labour, e.g. discovery of multiple pregnancy or malpresentation. Specialist care should be arranged during the confinement.
- Other women may have circumstances which increase risk;
  levels during pregnancy, e.g. heavy smokers, poor home circumstances;
  such women may need social support services in the community.
- Finally, some women may have a higher risk because of ethnic differences – antenatal care needs to be made acceptable to them.
- The antenatal plan agreed with women should allow involvement of the father whenever possible and a visit to the maternity unit where delivery is planned. Women should be clear about where parentcraft classes are available and the total number of antenatal visits (with GP or midwife) should be clarified and agreed.

30 marks

5. Record cards

These should allow recording of medical obstetric and social data, estimated date of delivery (EDD) and haematological investigation (rhesus factor, rubella status and blood group). It should also be possible to record preferred length of postnatal stay and the woman's wishes about mode of delivery and pain relief.

10 marks

6. Subsequent care

- Antenatal care for women whose pregnancies are progressing normally may be undertaken efficiently by the GP or the midwife as long as easy transfer to consultant care is available and there is full access to diagnostic facilities. There is a general under-utilization of midwives' skills.
- The reasons for procedures and tests and their results should be explained to all women who must be given the opportunity to decline them.
- Women who fail to attend clinics must be followed up. In any case, all women should be visited at home in early pregnancy to discuss arrangements and plans.

10 marks

7. The hospital service – priorities as seen from general practice

- Need for a small group of staff doing less but more high risk work.
- Need for antenatal pathology and pharmacy services to be near to each other.
- Need for realistic appointments system giving due regard to women's needs and avoiding long periods of waiting and overcrowding.
- Need for welcoming atmosphere, approachable staff, adequate seating and play area for children. Need for adequate refreshment and toilet facilities.
- Need for privacy during examination and an opportunity to build up a relationship of trust with a minimal number of staff who become known to the patient.

15 marks

10 discretionary marks

This is an unusual type of question which does test your understanding of the organizational and political aspects of the delivery of care and at the same time tests your understanding of the unique aspects of the work of the general practitioner.

Useful ideas may be obtained by reading: *Maternity Care In Action. A Guide to Good Practice and a Plan for Action.* Part 1. *Antenatal Care.* First Report of the Maternity Services Advisory Committee, DHSS, London, 1982.

Q2   A 22-year-old man presents with a 10-day history of 'indigestion' which has been eased to an extent by antacids. Discuss in detail your management plans and the principles which underline them.

A2   1. Introduction

- Heartburn, flatulence, nausea and epigastric discomfort are common problems in general practice. The general practitioner with 2500 patients will see each year: 50 patients with heartburn, flatulence and nausea; 40 patients with functional abdominal pain; 20 patients with functional constipation and diarrhoea; 30 or 40 patients with peptic ulcers.
- The natural history of duodenal ulcer is onset at 20–40 years of age with recurrent symptoms over 5–10 years and then spontaneous remission in as many as 60 per cent of cases.
- Major complications (bleeding and perforation) occur in 20 per cent of duodenal ulcers. A further 20 per cent of patients have chronic problems with severe and persistent symptoms; some in this group may require surgery.
- The peak age for gastric ulcer is 40–60 and virtually all patients with gastric carcinoma present over the age of 40.

15 marks

2. Assessment

- A careful history will determine what the patient means by indigestion, where it is, whether it is related to anything, what relieves it and whether he has noticed it before.
- There is a close relationship between indigestion and lifestyle. Enquiry would need to be made into smoking and drinking habits, employment and leisure, marital circumstances and life events.
- Why has the patient come? What is in his mind in view of the fact that he has had relief from antacids. Many patients worry about cancer. Perhaps there is a family history of 'ulcers'.
- The differential diagnosis lies between duodenal ulcer and 'non-ulcer dyspepsia'. Gastric ulcer is rare at this age and gastric cancer even rarer. Pancreatitis, cholecystitis and cardiac ischaemia are most unlikely.
- Physical examination is unlikely to provide further information after a careful history but may be helpful in reassuring the patient that his problems are being taken seriously, that he is being examined 'properly' and therefore may catalyse the development of a good history. Disadvantages include teaching the patient that an examination is 'necessary' when it isn't and that there might be something to find.

30 marks

3. Management

- It is not necessary to have a precise diagnosis before managing this patient. The differential diagnosis lies between duodenal ulceration and non-ulcer dyspepsia and management choices include further antacids along with lifestyle advice or an H_2-receptor antagonist.

- The case for antacids involves the fact that H_2-receptor antagonists are expensive and ideally should be prescribed only after a precise diagnosis has been made usually by endoscopy. The case for H_2-receptor antagonists involves the fact that they are very effective especially when symptoms have been prolonged or troublesome or recurrent. They need not necessarily be preceded by an endoscopy if care is taken in prescribing and in follow-up.
- A good approach (particularly if this patient was presenting for the very first time) would be to prescribe an antacid such as Asilone suspension with the following advice:

  i.   Take the antacid in appropriate dosages 4-hourly.
  ii. Do not follow any specific diet but avoid foods that aggravate the problem.
  iii. Eat small amounts of food frequently rather than large meals infrequently. This means breakfast and evening meal, mid-morning snack, lunch and mid-afternoon snack. Put time aside for this even if it is only a glass of milk and a biscuit. Rushing around is a sure way to aggravate indigestion.
  iv. Take the antacid between all these little meals so that there is always something in the stomach to counteract acidity and relieve symptoms.
  v.   Remember that smoking and alcohol can aggravate dyspepsia.
  vi. Return for follow-up if the problem does not settle down.

- If the patient returns fairly soon or presents with recurrent dyspepsia, a good approach would be to prescribe a month's treatment with cimetidine $400\,mg \times 2$ at night or ranitidine $150\,mg \times 2$ at night, and see the patient again. If symptoms have not settled down (or if they quickly recur after stopping therapy) referral for endoscopy is indicated.
- The patient should be aware of management plans for the future particularly if the natural history suggests duodenal ulceration. The development of surgical complications (haemorrhage, perforation, stenosis) are automatic indications for referral whether for surgery or blood transfusion. If episodes of pain are occurring several times a year despite H_2-receptor antagonists there may be no alternative to some form of vagotomy, preferably highly selective vagotomy.

45 marks

10 discretionary marks

Dyspepsia is a common practice presentation which inevitably brings in physical, psychological and social aspects of care. It also brings in the relationship between the GP and the patient and the GP and the hospital.

Q3   Write short notes on
A   Hysterectomy.
B   Migraine.

A3   **A. Hysterectomy**

1. A common problem

- The GP spends a lot of time with women whose symptoms may lead ultimately to hysterectomy. The act of referral increases the likelihood of surgery so it is crucial that the GP makes it crystal clear to the gynaecologist whether referral is to help the patient or the GP to cope, or to remove the uterus.
- In the average practice of 2500, 80 women are likely to have had a hysterectomy; by the age of 65, 14 per cent of women will have had a hysterectomy. Each year the GP or the team will be involved in counselling two women about the operation.
- Today most uteri are removed for benign disease. In 1975 in England and Wales: 7 per cent of hysterectomies were for malignancies of the genital tract; 33 per cent were for disorders of menstruation; 25 per cent were for fibroids; 12 per cent were for prolapse; 23 per cent were unclassified.
- It is significant that the age standardized hysterectomy rate is three times higher in the USA than in England and Wales. In the UK, hysterectomy rates vary widely across the regions, for example from 180 per 100 000 population at risk per annum in Mersey to about 290 per 100 000 in north-east Thames. In the Oxford region, there is a social class gradient the rate being twice as high in social class 1.

  ⋆ The reasons for these variations are complex and may not reflect disease but rather the perceptions of women themselves, the behaviour of their GPs and the views of their gynaecologists.

20 marks

2. The GP role

- The general practitioner and/or other team members must be prepared to discuss a number of issues with a woman considering hysterectomy.

  First, the need for the operation must be negotiated with the patient herself so that she is clear precisely what she is asking for. She must know exactly what will be removed and whether the ovaries will be left and whether the cervix will be removed. The GP must be familiar with the attitudes and practice of local gynaecologists.
- With regard to the question of whether or not the ovaries should be removed, some gynaecologists have set firm age limits, e.g. 45 years, beyond which they would always remove the ovaries at the time of hysterectomy because they may become malignant and it is argued that they serve no useful purpose. However, we do not know the long-term hormonal implications in older women as the ovaries do not in fact cease to have hormone-producing functions at the end of reproductive life.
- The possible psychological effects of hysterectomy require discussion. The position is contentious. One retrospective general practice study found that 37 per cent of 200 women who had a hysterectomy were treated for postoperative depression. Particularly vulnerable were women under 40 and those in whom there was no obvious pelvic pathology at hysterectomy; other factors included the presence of a

history of depression. However, more recent prospective hospital studies have not confirmed these findings.

- Many women have anxieties about sexual performance and libido after hysterectomy. There should be no such sequelae after uncomplicated surgery. Granulations of the vault can be treated with a silver nitrate stick. Atrophic vaginitis may denote declining oestrogen activity and may be treated with local oestrogen creams and systemic hormone therapy.

    Advice about when to resume full physical activity after surgery is best discussed with the individual patient as the usual advice of 6–8 weeks must vary enormously between different individuals.

30 marks

B. Migraine

1. Natural history and assessment

- Migraine is a common condition and very few patients require investigation or referral to hospital. Classic migraine hardly ever results from intracranial pathology. The differential diagnosis is usually between a tension headache and migraine attack. The former does not present with an aura or classic associated symptoms of nausea, vomiting and perhaps sensory or motor disturbances. Most patients are more ready to accept a diagnosis of migraine than tension headace.
- The symptom complex constituting migraine occurs in about 6 per cent of general practice patients and there is an annual prevalence rate of about 2 per cent. About 60 per cent develop the condition in their teens and early twenties and there is a period of activity of 10–15 years. Follow-up studies show that 40 per cent cease to suffer attacks over 25 years, in another 50 per cent attacks are well controlled and only 10 per cent of patients have an incapaciting problem.

    At any given time, 10 per cent of migraine victims are disabled by severe and frequent attacks, 30 per cent suffer an attack at least monthly with some disturbance to regular life and 60 per cent are only slightly inconvenienced by infrequent attacks which occur less than monthly and cause little interference to their regular life.
- Migraine sufferers tend to be tense, in the higher social classes and type 'A' personalities or 'go getters'.

    There is often a family history.
- Common trigger factors include stress, drugs (especially nitroglycerin, calcium, antagonists, hydralazine and aminophylline), alcohol, hormones and certain foods (cheese, chocolate, fried food, onion, citrus fruits).

25 marks

2. Management

- Management includes patient education about the nature of the condition and the benefits and limitations of treatment. The patient should be encouraged to avoid trigger factors and stressful situations.

A mild attack may well respond to a simple analgesic such as aspirin or paracetamol taken early in the attack. An antiemetic such as metoclopramide (Maxolon) may be helpful in a dose of 5–10 mg three times daily.

A severe attack may need rest in a darkened room and an ergot preparation. Prophylactic treatment may be necessary. A useful drug is pizotifen (Sanomigran) in a dose of 1.5–6.0 mg daily in divided doses. An alternative would be clonidine (Dixarit) 50–75 mg twice daily or propranolol 10–20 mg twice daily.

- Relaxation therapy is claimed to help in about 80 per cent of patients.
- Some patients would benefit from joining a Migraine Society and reading their literature. Self-care is an important concept to introduce.

25 marks

This question contains two parts: one problem automatically involves a hospital consultant in management, the second usually doesn't.

The hysterectomy question needs to concentrate on the GP's role which will have much to do with negotiating the need for the operation, explaining what will happen and providing aftercare. The migraine question will need to cover diagnostic criteria and management options.

A useful source of information for all aspects of gynaecology in general practice is: *Women's Problems in General Practice*, edited by A. McPherson and A. Anderson, Oxford, Oxford University Press, 1983.

PTQ
TEST 2

Answers

Q1 *'The Medical Profession has become a major threat to health.'*
Ivan Illich, 1977

Discuss your reaction to this statement with special reference to the role of the general practitioner.

A1 **1. Preamble**

In order to react to this statement at all it is essential to define 'health' in some way.

There are many 'definitions' ranging from 'an absence of disease' to a 'continuing perfect adjustment of an organism to its environment'. No definition is universally agreed.

10 marks

2. Arguments supporting Illich

Basically the arguments reflect undercare and overcare at the interface between the GP and the community and between the GP and the hospital or secondary service.

- The economic arguments: the potential cost of health care is unlimited. Its cost is rising everywhere partly as a result of new technology, partly as a result of the increasing presentation of psychosocial problems which are 'medicalized' by GPs, e.g. the use of benzodiazepines for anxiety, and partly because medicalizing acute self-limiting illness takes away the ability of people to look after themselves.
- The iatrogenesis argument: overprescribing is a demonstrable problem in general practice. Even when we don't prescribe, our behaviour teaches patients to buy 'over-the-counter' remedies. On any given day, 60 per cent of the population are taking drugs. Drugs have harmful as well as beneficial effects.
- There is evidence of undercare in general practice. The Black Report presents an argument that, despite 40 years of a National Health Service, we have failed to tackle effectively the health imbalance between rich and poor. Patients in lower social classes die earlier, have more morbidity and more accidents.
- Another example of undercare in general practice is the relative neglect of patients with chronic illness, e.g. half our hypertensives are undiagnosed and, even when they are diagnosed and on treatment, half are poorly controlled.
- At the interface with the hospital there is evidence of late referral of many patients with cancer and over-referral of other patients (such as late-onset diabetics) who might best be cared for in general practice. Referral habits of GPs (and their cost to the community) vary by as much as a factor of 10.

139

- A final argument could be a global attack on primary care which, for example, in the less developed countries has failed to provide for rural communities and has concentrated its attention on a minority of people in the cities, often providing inappropriate high technology Western-style medicine.

30 marks

3. Arguments defending general practice

- Simply caring: the public (as evidenced by frequent questionnaires) values highly the existence of the personal and caring support (whether physical, psychological or social) provided by the GP at a time of crisis. This support is highly regarded and beneficial almost irrespective of the outcome, e.g. terminal care.
- Immunization: although social change accounts for a large part of the reduction in impact of the infectious diseases, immunization has played its part. The dramatic fall in the level of protection in the under-fives against whooping cough after the 'scares' of the seventies resulted in a major recurrence of this disease. Rubella, measles and poliomyelitis etc. are other examples.
- Health education: the potential in general practice for health education is enormous in terms of persuading people to abandon unhealthy lifestyles. Many people will readily admit that they lost weight, stopped smoking or drinking too much alcohol because of the intervention of a GP who they respected.
- Cervical cytology programmes are another example of the GP's role in prevention. Most cervical smears are carried out by GPs.
- GPs are also taking over the care of chronic illness from hospitals. Diabetic clinics in general practice are an example of this.
- General practitioners have an influence on the care delivered in hospitals. Improvement in the obstetric services demanded by women, for example, have been catalysed by the intervention of GPs.

30 marks

30 discretionary marks

Discretionary marks would be awarded for clarity of argument and the development of a 'balanced' view.

This is essentially a question about the advantages and disadvantages of medical care. No human system, however well intentioned, can be 'risk' or 'side effect' free and the examiner is looking for a well argued grasp of the problems involved. Although Illich's statement is provocative, the marking schedule will allow for different reactions to occur either supporting Illich, attacking him or presenting a 'balanced' response.

Helpful reading

1. For definitions of health: Lee, P. R. and Franks, P. E. (1980) Health and disease in the community. In *Primary Care*, edited by John Fry. Heinemann, London
2. Illich, I. (1977) *Medical Nemesis. The Expropriation of Health.* Penguin Books, London

Q2   *Discuss in detail the childhood immunization programme, including the contraindications to the various vaccines.*
   In practice, how would you try to achieve the highest uptake rates possible?

A2   **1. Preamble**

Although social change accounts for most of the dramatic improvement in the mortality and morbidity of the common infective diseases during the last century, immunization has played a significant part. The dramatic fall in the level of protection in under-fives after the over-publicized 'scares' about pertussis vaccine in the '70s led to a major recurrence of whooping cough.

A rational and well balanced practice programme should result in over 90 per cent being effectively immunized. How easy this is to achieve will reflect the social class make-up of the practice as the upper social classes are both easier to convince of the value of immunization and are more ready to attend. In this instance, good clinical practice will be good business practice and the item of service rewards boost practice income.

10 marks

2. Vaccine programme

Diphtheria, pertussis and tetanus vaccine (triple vaccine) is usually administered at 3, 4½ and 6½–11 months together with oral polio vaccine. In the event of a whooping cough epidemic, can give 'crash' course of three doses of triple at monthly intervals from 3 months. Booster doses of tetanus and diphtheria should be given at 12–18 months, if this regimen is used. Prematurely born infants should be immunized at the usual chronological age.

Infants whose basic courses have been interrupted should be given a single additional dose later in infancy (or two doses where only the first dose of the basic course has been given) regardless of the time elapsing between the initial and subsequent doses. A preschool booster of diphtheria/tetanus and polio should be given at 4½ years.

Measles vaccine is given in the second year (not earlier than 15 months) and rubella at 10 years to girls. In 1988 this regimen will be replaced by a new vaccine, MMR, which contains measles, mumps and rubella. This will be administered during the second year of life. The programme is completed by receiving booster of diphtheria, tetanus vaccine and oral polio before school entry.

BCG is given at birth to certain ethnic groups, particularly from the Indian subcontinent and refugees from South-East Asia. BCG is still generally recommended for 11- to 13-year-olds who are Heaf test negative although some authorities are abandoning the practice.

An opportunity exists for the general practitioner to identify 'high' risk and 'low' risk children in his practice and immunize accordingly.

25 marks

3. Contraindications to vaccines

For all practical purposes, in children there are no contraindications to diphtheria and tetanus vaccine/toxoid. Absolute contraindications to pertussis are acute febrile illness (postpone until recovered), history of a severe local or general reaction to a previous dose, history of cerebral irritation or damage in the neonatal period and the infant suffering from fits. Relative contraindications are parents or siblings with idiopathic epilepsy, child with neurological diseases or developmental delay thought to be due to neurological defect.

Live vaccines (polio, measles, rubella) should not be given to children on oral steroids or immunosuppressant therapy or to those suffering from malignant disease or immunological dysfunction. Acute febrile illness should lead to postponement until recovered.

Specific contraindications to polio immunization are diarrhoea and vomiting (postpone until recovered) and past history of serious adverse reaction to penicillin. To measles are active TB and history of anaphylactoid reaction to egg ingestion; personal or family history of fits is not a contraindication to measles vaccination and such children should be vaccinated with simultaneous administration of dilute human normal immunoglobulin. To rubella are thrombocytopenia and rheumatoid arthritis.

BCG should not be given at site of local septic conditions or at site of chronic skin disease or to children with Heaf positive reactions (except grade 1).

25 marks

4. Practice procedures

- The immunization programme should be discussed with the parents early, starting during antenatal visits. The programme should be discussed again at postnatal visits, so that a firm decision to immunize can be agreed by 6 weeks. Midwives and health visitors should participate in this programme.
- Anxieties, whether real or imagined, can be managed at these times remembering that some patients may be reluctant to voice them.
- The practice may choose to send out it's own 'reminders' or allow the FPC computer to do this. The program could be managed by the health visitors or the practice nurse. Local authority nurses may be reluctant to involve themselves.
- The product information expiry dates of the vaccine and any possible contraindication must be checked before any patient is given vaccine. It is particularly important that every practice should have available the DHSS circular (31 March 1977) on precautions to be observed before carrying out immunization procedures. There must be facilities to cope with an anaphylactic reaction – 1:1000 adrenaline is not sufficient. Intravenous hydrocortisone, chlorpheniramine 10 mg i.v. and intravenous fluids and a Brooks' airway and oxygen cylinder should be readily available.
- If there is a practice nurse, she should be allowed to vaccinate 'all comers' whenever she is working. If the GPs do their own immunizing, then they should be prepared to vaccinate whenever feasible.
- Must have some system to identify non-attenders and to allow health visitors to follow them up.
- It is good practice for the primary health care team to send out reminders for the measles vaccination programme in the second year of life, and to send for 10-year-old girls, e.g. by birthday card and letter on their tenth birthday, before the schools programme begins at 11 years. Patients can be identified from the age–sex register or a specific card index.

Quite apart from the income produced, an active approach to immunization demonstrates a 'caring' approach which helps to maintain the doctor–patient relationship. Do not forget that opportunistic immunization (e.g. measles) can be given when children attend for other reasons, provided the clinical records allow the doctor to 'see' what the child has missed, e.g. if back of Lloyd George envelope is reserved solely to record immunizations given, then can be scanned by GP easily at any consultation with a child.

30 marks

10 discretionary marks

> This question assesses not only our knowledge of immunization routines, including contraindications to vaccines, but also your ideas about implementing a successful programme in your practice.

Q3 *A 70-year-old man presents with a 3-month history of hesitancy, nocturia, slowness of the urine stream and terminal dribbling.*
     Discuss in detail how you would care for this patient indicating the likely diagnosis.

A3 ## 1. Introduction

The symptoms suggest 'outflow obstruction', the likely cause being benign prostatic hypertrophy which is an almost inevitable consequence of ageing.

- The prevalence in men over 40 is at least 80 per cent.
- A man aged 40 has a 10 per cent chance of requiring prostatic surgery if he lives to the age of 80.
- Four per cent of men over 80 need prostatectomy.

10 marks

2. Assessment

Involves a multitude of factors.

- Is this outflow obstruction? The history is crucial. The earliest symptoms suggesting bladder neck obstruction must be identified and differentiated from symptoms such as burning and frequency which suggests infection. Is there any evidence to suggest diabetes, multiple sclerosis, cord compression or drug side effects (e.g. anticholinergics)?
- Psychological and social circumstances are very important. Does the patient live alone? Is he incontinent and does he require help with washing facilities? Can the district nurse or social services be of any help? Decisions about surgery may well be influenced by the effect of 'wetting and incontinence' on those who look after the patient.

- Physical examination should include the abdomen (bladder enlargement) and rectal examination (prostate enlargement may be malignant – areas of induration may be felt) and a neurological examination of the lower limbs if a neurogenic bladder is suspected. Men with mild symptoms can be in retention.
- Some investigations can be carried out from general practice, e.g. mid-stream specimen of urine (MSSU) and intravenous pyelogram (IVP) (which helps to give information about residual urine, trabeculation of the bladder and hypertrophy) – all providing objective evidence of the *degree* of outflow obstruction.

30 marks

3. Management

- Once it is clear that the patient has bladder neck obstruction (as opposed to prostatism or urinary tract infection) the emphasis in general practice is on early referral and consultant assessment so that information about the degree of obstruction can be titrated against the patient's own ideas allowing a decision to be made about surgery. Acute or chronic retention must be avoided if at all possible in order to preserve renal function, but the quality of the patient's life is no less important.
- There are three possible attitudes towards the patient who has symptoms or obstruction – he can put up with it, he can have a prostatectomy or he can wear a catheter. Patients tend to fall into two groups as a result of these considerations.

Group one
For these patients the choice lies between a permanent indwelling catheter and prostatectomy; the advice to put up with it is unthinkable. They tend to be men who present in acute or chronic retention, have severe symptoms and haematuria and who, on investigation, already have renal failure, signs of upper tract obstruction or bladder trabeculation with diverticulae formation, and a considerable residual urine.

Group two
For these patients the choice lies between prostatectomy and putting up with it – a permanent indwelling catheter is unthinkable. They may have minimal symptoms, a residual urine below 60 ml and none of the above problems.

- The GP's advice should be based on several observations. Group one patients are easy as there are very few contraindications to surgery – if the patient is not entirely demented the operation is feasible. The only situation in which a catheter might be advised is in terminal illness. Group two patients can be more difficult. Many improve if nothing is done yet others present years later with severe back pressure effects.
- Relevant information includes the following when helping the patient to make up his mind:

    i. Prostatectomy is not necessarily a safe and reliable operation with a trivial mortality; it depends on who is doing it (urologist or general surgeon) and what type of operation is performed.
    ii. Transurethral prostatectomy is as reliable and as effective as transvesical prostatectomy and is significantly safer in terms of morbidity and mortality. It also requires a shorter period of hospital admission.
    iii. High risk cases are patients over the age of 80, those with an associated diagnosis not involving the urinary tract and those admitted as an emergency in retention.

- It is the GP's responsibility to organize adequate follow-up when patients do not receive surgery to identify deteriorating symptoms and urinary tract infection. A second opinion may become necessary.
- The usual result of a modern prostatectomy is a satisfied patient who is able to leave hospital within a week or 10 days passing uninfected urine with good control and a good stream. He should be able to return to normal activities within 3 weeks and, of course, he may golf, garden or pursue his usual hobbies. Sexual intercourse is possible as soon as the patient returns home, although retrograde ejaculation may occur. Continuing symptoms may mean the incomplete removal of an adenoma and carcinoma may develop in the outer (surgical) capsule of the gland as may a further adenoma. Myocardial infarct and pulmonary embolism are the commonest causes of death complicating surgery. The commonest non-fatal complication is a degree of incontinence (more likely in the older patient) which may respond to perineal faradism.

50 marks

10 discretionary marks

This is a typical example of a question selected from the area of clinical practice. When preparing your answer remember that problem definition and management will need to reflect the work of the GP rather than pathophysiology and hospital care, and therefore the emphasis will need to be on the former rather than the lattter.

Q1 *Discuss the ways in which the general practitioner, the district nurse and the health visitor might cooperate in the delivery of primary health care. Indicate your preferences giving reasons for your choice.*

A1 **1. Introduction**

- The primary health care needs of the community (prevention, diagnosis, management, education) are so complex that no one individual discipline can possibly cope. Doctors and nurses therefore have no choice but to cooperate in the delivery of that care – willingly or not.
- These health care needs are changing rapidly. For example:
  - i. Acute infections are being replaced by chronic degenerative diseases.
  - ii. Unemployment and marital strife are transmuted into problems that are presented at primary care level. This means that not only must doctors and nurses work together, but they must do so flexibly, particularly if primary health care is to be both effective and economic.
- There is a need to shift professional behaviour from professional control towards patient participation and self-care. This means new skills to enable unhealthy populations to change their lifestyles.

10 marks

2. Ways of working together

- There are four possible modes of employment of team members:
  - i. Employment by the DHA for all team members.
  - ii. Independent contractor (self-employed) status for all team members.
  - iii. Employment of a member of one discipline by another (e.g. practice nurse).
  - iv. A mixed system within one team (as at present in the UK).
- There are two ways in which team members can deliver care:
  - i. From the same premises.
  - ii. From separate premises.
- There are two ways in which team members can share patient care:
  - i. Working separately in order to solve problem and then communicating.
  - ii. Working together to identify and then solve problems.
- Teams require leadership and discipline. This can be exercised in two basic ways:
  - i. When discipline is exerted from outside the team.

    ii. When discipline is exerted from within the team: one member is seen as having more authority than another, or leadership is seen as having more to do with team direction and function (like small group leadership) than it has with telling other professionals what to do and how to do it.

30 marks

3. Comment

- With regard to the mode of employment, team function is likely to be optimum when all team members are employed the same way (e.g. reflect on the resulting problems when DHA nurses are seen as earning money for independent contractor GPs).
- If nurses work in a nursing hierarchy, the result is that nurses by joining together, achieve more power and independence from GPs, but an undesirable consequence is that a nursing hierarchy impedes the development of nursing by resisting the introduction of new nursing tasks. Nurses are told what they may and may not do without regard to their ability to do it.
- Employment of a nurse by a doctor may ease care problems (as a doctor sees them for example) but an employed nurse is a controlled nurse however liberal the employer. The pressures will be 'to instruct' or 'to allow' rather than for the nurse to decide for herself.
- The 'independent contractor' nurse would have freedom and independence to develop her discipline and this might be to the advantage of society (rapid response to changing needs and care delivered economically), but relatively few nurses may want the commitment.
- Working from separate premises cannot make for more effective teamwork. The concept of a registered practice population allows for closer ties with a community than a concept of a 'neighbourhood population' (Cumberledge) which allows less choice for the patient and would be counterproductive unless GPs joined it.
- Optimum team effectiveness would depend on the ability to work separately (in the individual professional consultation) and together (e.g. defining and managing a problem list for a family with a member who has a stroke) as the occasion demanded.
- Hierarchies – whether operating within a team (e.g. the practice nurse) or outside the team (e.g. nurse management) – slow down the response to changing community need. The ideal has to be independent contractor status for all who look after a registered practice population with leadership having to do with team effectiveness and function and direction. Money earned could be distributed to each member of the team according to the value of the work done and training and skills would determine that. A difficulty is not all nurses would want this. An alternative might be a salaried service for all.

    The difficulty is few GPs would want this.

40 marks

20 discretionary marks

Team care is an important concept at the present time. The candidate must be prepared to argue why and demonstrate an understanding of why different disciplines have difficulty working together.

This question requires the ability to write down the theoretical ways in which nurses and doctors can work together and argue the advantages and disadvantages of each.

Q2 *Discuss the ways in which the practice might improve its performance in caring for patients who drink alcohol.*

A2 **1. Preamble**

- The amount of alcohol we drink reflects society's attitudes towards drinking. Individual patients (and doctors) also have beliefs about the amount of alcohol that can be drunk without giving rise to a problem.
- The harm which alcohol can inflict is directly related to consumption in the individual. In recent years we have derived guidelines (which may or may not be accurate) about the amount of alcohol (units per day or per week) below which there should be no problem. This means that old concepts such as alcohol addiction or problem drinking may not be our only cause for concern.
- The harm resulting from drinking alcohol may be physical, psychological or social and the amount of alcohol we consume has increased. We drink twice as much now as we did in 1950 and women have contributed to this increase.

15 marks

2. Recognition, recording assessment

- Many practices obtain clinical and social data about newly registered patients either by appointments, general questionnaire or by interview with a nurse.
- Screening projects are formidable to undertake and 'opportunistic' screening during other consultations is more practicable.
- There are 'high risk' factors for heavy drinking (e.g. family history, certain occupations) and these patients should be 'targetted' in any practice screening programme.

15 marks

3. Programme for action

- A unit for alcohol is a half pint of beer, a glass of wine or a single measure of spirits. Patients can be divided into three categories:

  i. Patients who drink little or no alcohol (women 15 units or under weekly – men 20 units or under weekly).
  ii. Patients who have a high consumption (women above 35 units weekly – men above 50 units weekly).
  iii. Moderate drinkers – those with an intermediate pattern.

A practice with 2000 patients might have only 40 men and 15 women in the high risk category, but would have 140 men and 77 women who are moderate drinkers.

High risk patients should be advised to reduce consumption and should be monitored closely. Moderate drinkers should be warned that, according to our current ideas, they could be at risk and should be reviewed annually. Others should be reviewed every 5 years.

It should be remembered that the very young, the pregnant and very old are more at risk and there may be additive or synergistic factors such as chronic illness, certain drugs and psychological conditions. Some patients may have a low consumption and a high vulnerability.

25 marks

4. Offering help

i. *High risk patients*
    The aim must be to reduce consumption. Patients may be ready to act, they may understand the problem but not be ready to act or they may not have thought about their drinking at all.

    Patients ready to act – such patients need advice on 'how to do it', e.g. taking smaller sips, taking rest days, learning how to refuse. Referral may be necessary to other team members (e.g. clinical psychologists, AA community alcohol teams, detoxication units).

    - Patients who understand the problems need help in decision making weighing up and altering the balance sheet in terms of the good and harmful effects of drinking.
    - Patients who have not thought about their drinking need to understand the relationship between drinking and harm and why the doctor is worried even if the patient isn't. Keeping a drinking diary can help as can identifying problems related to drinking. Blood tests may provide evidence of damage, e.g. macrocytosis, elevated gammaglutamyl transferase.

ii. *Moderate risk patients*
    May have a high or low vulnerability to the effects of alcohol. If the patient is not vulnerable advice is necessary to reduce consumption below 20 units for men and 15 units for women each week. Education can include:

    - Presenting a summary of the assessment findings (consumption, current effects on health, evidence of tolerance).
    - Discussion of laboratory tests and their reversibility.
    - Indicate patients position on a consumption histogram.

    Follow-up appointments should be negotiated with these patients.

iii. *Minimal risk patients*
     Need no further action other than the awareness that vulnerability can change.

30 marks

15 discretionary marks

Remember that 'the practice' consists of people (patients and professionals) who work in a care delivery system (premises and programmes) which may be good or bad.

Do not forget that 'care for' includes treatment, prevention and education. *RCGP Report from General Practice No. 24 1986, *Alcohol – a Balanced View*, is a good source of information.

* Note that there is no mention of alcohol addiction or problem drinking – the question states patients who drink alcohol.

Q3 *Write short notes on:*
A *Vertigo.*
B *Frozen shoulder.*

A3 ## A. Vertigo

1. Preamble

- Patients do not complain of vertigo. They complain of dizziness or loss of balance. Dizziness is a vague term and may mean little more than a light-headed or woolly sensation in the head. Vertigo is an illusion of movement in the individual or the environment; the patient himself or objects around him appear to spin. There is always a sense of movement. However, although vertigo is always associated with imbalance, imbalance is not always due to vertigo.
  Vertigo may be central, intermediate (vestibular nerve) or peripheral.
- Central causes include tumour, epilepsy, multiple sclerosis, head injury, infection, benign positional vertigo and vascular disturbances. About 10 per cent of cases are psychogenic.
  Intermediate causes include vestibular neuronitis, acoustic neuroma and ototoxic drugs. Peripheral causes include Menière's disease, labyrinthitis, head injury with temporal bone fracture and vascular inner ear disturbance.

15 marks

2. Assessment

- The approach in the consulting room must begin by establishing by careful history that the problem is in fact vertigo, its duration, frequency and severity. The next step is to rule out systemic causes or extralabyrinthine causes needing urgent investigation, such as destructive middle ear disease or any central vestibular abnormality. The ears must be examined carefully and any wax removed. The gait can be observed and Romberg's test (which assesses stance) can be carried out with the eyes open and closed.
- Nystagmus may be of central origin when there are other neurological symptoms and signs when the story does not fit into one of the peripheral labyrinthine patterns and when spontaneous jerk nystagmus has central features or when positionally provoked nystagmus (Hallpike's test) is associated with other neurological abnormalities and persists.

15 marks

2. Menière's disease

- About 10 per cent of patients with vertigo have Menière's disease. It is a disease of the young and middle-aged and is rare after the age of 50. Attacks are characterized by violent paroxysmal vertigo associated with deafness and tinnitus. Nausea and vomiting are common. Vasodilator drugs include betahistine (Serc) 8 mg three times daily; nicotinic acid 25–50 mg three times daily is a useful alternative. Labyrinthine sedatives such as prochlorperazine (Stemetil 5 g) should be reserved for the acute attacks. Twenty per cent of patients require surgery.

10 marks

4. Benign paroxysmal vertigo

- Benign paroxysmal (positional) vertigo is a common problem provoked by movements of the head, usually to one side when turning in bed or on looking upwards. Each attack lasts only a few seconds in contrast to Menière's disease in which an attack may last 2–3 hours. There is usually no obvious cause but the problem may follow a trivial head injury. Reassurance is an important part of management.

5 marks

5. Other causes

- Vertebrobasilar ischaemia and cervical vertigo tend to coexist. In pure cervical spondylosis, osteophytes press on posterior rami of the upper cervical nerve roots carrying proprioceptive impulses to the vestibular nuclei. In pure vertebrobasilar ischaemia osteophytes press on vertebral arteries. A cervical collar is helpful.

5 marks

B. Frozen shoulder

1. Preamble

- The glenohumeral joint is surrounded by a 'rotator cuff' which blends into the joint capsule. It consists of the combined tendons of the subscapularis supraspinatus, infraspinatus and teres minor. In addition, the long head of the biceps arises inside the capsule of the joint and leaves it alongside the bicipital groove in the humerus passing through a small foramen in the joint capsule.
- Although it is well known that pain in the shoulder can be referred from elsewhere, notably the neck, lungs, heart and diaphragm, these sources are relatively rare as are degenerative arthropathies of the glenohumeral or acromioclavicular joints. In over 90 per cent of patients, shoulder pain is caused by the rotator cuff syndrome/capsulitis group of lesions. The rotator cuff, and particularly the supraspinatus tendon, commonly undergoes a focal necrosis, which may progress to a generalized chronic inflammation of the whole rotator cuff mechanism and joint capsule. Fibrosis and adhesive capsulitis may then ensue and the outcome is a stiff but painless frozen shoulder.
- The pathogenesis is largely obscure but the peak incidence is between 50 and 70 years of age and women are affected rather more than men. Onset may be spontaneous but it may be associated with arm immobilization following stroke, thoracic surgery, myocardial infarction and cervical herpes zoster. Other factors include trauma to the shoulder from sports injuries or manual work.

15 marks

2. Assessment

• The usual presentation is shoulder pain, often worse at night with cuff tenderness and a painful arc on abduction which indicates supraspinatus involvement. There may be loss of passive rotation of the arm (all movements at the glenohumeral joint) and crepitus, which could signify adhesive capsulitis. However, the most important sign differentiating the rotator cuff syndrome from adhesive capsulitis is pain on attempted abduction and/or external rotation of the dependent arm against resistance. Shoulder pain on resisted internal rotation indicates subscapularis tendinitis and on resisted supination and flexion of the forearm it implies bicipital tendinitis. Clinical assessment should also include movements of the cervical spine, to exclude referred pain, and inspection for joint swellings and signs of arthritis.

15 marks

3. Management

• As the process is usually self-limiting after a year or two, it has been notoriously difficult to assess the value of active treatment, and this remains controversial. The usual management involves mobilizing physiotherapy, short-wave diathermy and intra-articular injection of local steroids. Patients can be shown how to swing the arm to and fro like a simple pendulum in the sagittal plane and then to try a progressively larger arc using a stirring motion until a 360 degree vertical arc can be described. Oral non-steroidal anti-inflammatory drugs in full dosage should be prescribed.
• Many GPs have been reluctant to inject steroids into joint cavities presumably because of the possibility of infection. In practice this is most unlikely if sensible precautions are taken, such as swabbing the skin and using sterile needles and syringes.
   The choice of steroid has been between hydrocortisone acetate 20 mg/ml, which is ideal for mild lesions, and the more potent and longer acting methylprednisolone acetate (Depo-Medrone) 40 mg/ml, and triamcinolone hexacetonide (Lederspan) 20 mg/ml, which are used in smaller volumes. Under normal circumstances 1 ml methylprednisolone acetate is best combined with 1 ml lignocaine (1% plain). Half can be injected laterally into the shoulder joint and half by the anterior approach. A 2 ml syringe with a 1.5-inch (38-mm) needle is adequate. The patients should be warned that increased pain is likely for the first 48 hours after injection but that the pain should settle afterwards.

20 marks

Q1 Discuss the value of screening for hypertension in general practice. How should case findings be conducted and patients then managed?

A1 1. Preamble

- In order to justify a screening programme for anything, the following conditions should be satisfied:
  - i.   There must be an important disease.
  - ii.   There must be an accepted treatment.
  - iii. Facilities for diagnosis and treatment must be available.
  - iv.   There must be a latent (early symptomatic) stage.
  - v.   There must be a suitable test.
  - vi.   The test must be acceptable to the patients.
  - vii. The natural history of the disease must be understood.
  - viii. There must be an agreed policy on who to treat.
  - ix.   There must be a balance between case finding costs, treatment costs and patient community benefit.
  - x.   Case finding programmes must be continuous.

- Hypertension is worth screening for because:
  - i.   At any time 10–15 per cent of the population have a blood pressure >160/90. The risk of complications and death are directly related to BP levels. Complications include strokes, heart failure, sudden heart attack, kidney damage, eye damage. Treatment may be urgent if BP >250/140, if there is target organ damage, if the patient is young or if there is a bad family history.
  - ii.   There are many acceptable forms of treatment.
  - iii. Facilities for diagnosis and treatment are readily available in the GP surgery. Case finding is best conducted on an opportunistic basis as 95 per cent of the GP population will see him over 5 years. Formal screening programmes are inordinately expensive. Only about 50 per cent of patients will respond to call or recall letters to attend screening procedures.
  - iv.   Most patients with high blood pressure are asymptomatic.
  - v.   Sphygomanometer readings are easily obtained and acceptable to patients.
  - vi.   Most hypertension (90–95 per cent) is essentially of unknown cause. Although the majority of hypertensives have normal life expectancies with no complications, high blood pressure doubles the risk of premature death (before age 70). Death rates from strokes are three times those of the whole population and treatment reduces this. Although malignant hypertension is rare (>250/140 – less than 5 per cent of all cases), if untreated causes death usually within a year.

vii. By and large *persistent* hypertension (three or more readings) >160/100–110 needs treatment.

viii. As long as the criteria considered under this section are followed, costs are balanced.

ix. Case finding is continuous if it is opportunistic in the GP surgery. Practices could reasonably agree to record a BP once every 5 years (if normal) in all 35- to 65-year-olds.

50 marks

2. Management

- All patients who are identified as hypertensives should be entered into a disease register and should have a special hypertension record card in their notes. All adult patients who are normotensive should have their blood pressure measured every 5 years.
- Urgent treatment is needed for patients with BP >250/140 mmHg, grade 4 retinopathy and uraemia, patients with target organ damage (heart, brain, kidneys).
- With lesser degrees of BP (diastolic 95–110 mmHg) factors suggesting treatment are young patients (<50 years), male patients, bad family history. Other adverse factors include high cholesterol, intractable smoking and diabetes.
- General measures include:

  i.   Control of other risk factors (smoking, stop Pill).
  ii. Reduce weight if obese.
  iii. Reduce salt intake.
  iv. Reduce alcohol intake.

- Specific treatment includes:

  i.   Diuretics.
  ii. Beta-blockers.
  iii. Peripheral vasodilators.
  iv. Others, e.g. methyldopa.

- Resistant hypertensives may need specialist advice; ? secondary hypertension.
- Follow-up (using disease register) can be managed by a community nurse or a practice nurse with agreed circumstances in which the doctor must be consulted. Stable hypertensives can be seen two or three times each year. A prescription can be given to cover this period. Alternatively a monitored repeat prescription system must be devised.

40 marks

10 discretionary marks

The question tests:

- Your knowledge of the value of screening.
- Your understanding of the natural history of hypertension.
- Your knowledge of management options.
- Your ability to organize care.

Q2   *Write short notes on:*
A   *Bedwetting.*
B   *Patient participation groups.*

A2   ## A. Bedwetting

1. Preamble

- Most children achieve control of bladder function during the day by the age of 3 years and at night by the age of 4 years. Dryness is a natural development which, like walking, emerges in the absence of training at an age determined by predisposing genetic factors; the latter can be influenced by environmental factors. Enuresis is common and there are interesting geographical and cultural variations, for example:

  i.   Ten per cent of all children are still wetting the bed occasionally on school entry.
  ii. Five per cent of children (more boys than girls) are still bedwetting at the age of 11 years.
  ii. At 14 years 1 per cent of boys and about 0.5 per cent of girls are still regularly wetting the bed.
  iv. In Sweden, about 8 per cent of 5-year-old children wet the bed at night. In Australia and North America the figure is about 20 per cent.
  v.   Bedwetting is commoner in social classes 4 and 5 and in overcrowded homes.

- Negative environmental factors that delay normal genetically determined maturation of bladder control mechanisms include separation from mother, a broken home, forceful 'potty training' and other stressful events in the second and third years of life.

10 marks

2. Assessment

- Although a preschool child will not be bothered about bedwetting (unless the mother is) a 6-year-old may be embarrassed, particularly if there are 'accidents' during the day as well and if he or she should be invited to spend a night with a school friend. The child should be given a chance to express his feelings. Usually at this age, however, the mother's feelings are paramount and one should ask whether wetting is a solitary symptom or one among others such as mild dysuria and/or frequency, listlessness and abdominal pain, which could suggest urinary tract infection.

  One should ask the mother about family norms for the attainment of dryness, including the ages at which it was achieved in grandparents, aunts, uncles and siblings. If maturational delay is demonstrated or secondary enuresis (after dryness has been attained) is the problem, precipitating causes should be explored. Is there stress at home or at school? What is the mother's attitude towards toilet training? How does she react when she finds a wet bed? Is she well herself? One should look at the family records, as the child's problem may well reflect a family disorder.

- A physical examination is unlikely to reveal positive physical signs, but is expected by the mother and will certainly be reassuring. Examination of the external genitalia in boys is probably worthwhile, for conditions such as hypospadias. Further investigation should be limited to the examination of a urine specimen for proteinuria, glycosuria and bacteriuria, although infection in children with wetting as a sole symptom is rare. There is no place for excretion urography.

15 marks

3. Management

- The most important aspect of management has by now already occurred, namely allowing the child and parent to discuss their views with a professional who has explained to them the process of attaining dryness. In many instances this may be enough, and children can be told that even if nothing further is done they will have more and more dry beds simply because they are growing up.

    Other families may need more support. Bedwetting is a risk factor for child abuse. A hard-pressed mother, depressed, with a low income and large family may need support from the social services, which could include the facilities of the borough laundry service.
- If a child has an important social event looming near, or if his mother was at her 'wits end', one should consider a temporary (2–3 week) prescription for imipramine syrup (Tofranil) 25–50 mg at night. There is often a satisfactory response but the relapse rate is high.
- By far the most effective and specific treatment is the use of the buzzer alarm, which can be used in suitably intelligent children down to the age of 5 years. The child sleeps on a detector mechanism such as mesh or foil mats connected to an alarm buzzer. The principle is conditioned learning, the mechanism being triggered by voided urine that completes the electrical circuit; the alarm wakens the child who gets out of bed to turn off the alarm and goes to the toilet. At first the bed is very wet before the child awakens thoroughly to the alarm, but with continued use he will awaken earlier and the wet patches will become smaller and smaller. Eventually he will awaken before the alarm goes (before he is wet) or will sleep through the night without needing to micturate.
- Most children will become dry within 4 months, usually in the first 2 months; the usual number of wet beds (with the buzzer) before dryness is 15–20. A success rate of 85 per cent with a relapse rate of only 10 per cent is claimed. Technical problems include false alarms and failure of the alarm to sound when the child wets – these can be tackled using the manufacturer's instructions.
- Children who fail to respond to treatment are a small but important group who require special management. The commonest reason is misuse of the buzzer apparatus, in which case the whole problem should be reassessed as above. There may well be no alternative to telling the child and the parents that the child's bladder is not yet ready to be dry. Referral to a paediatric colleague may be necessary if urinary incontinence is suspected (usually caused by spina bifida) or if the parents are becoming restive.

25 marks

B. Patient participation groups

1. Preamble

- The concept of patient participation has made much progress in recent years. The movement originated in the early 1970s when several GPs, acting independently, encouraged the formation of practice groups to consider health care problems. Although there are only about 30 known groups in existence, a national association was formed in 1978 after several groups had published their experiences. The Association now receives a DHSS grant towards headquarter's expenses, holds national conferences, organizes regional meetings and publishes a regular newsletter.

- No doubt patient groups are a product of the consumer-orientated age we live in, but other factors are relevant. All groups seem to depend crucially on the enthusiasm of one or more GPs who, although superficially different in terms of personal or background characteristics, share similar attitudes about health and towards general practice. They take the view that health is a great deal more than the absence of illness, disability or stress and that there is more to general practice than simply ameliorating these conditions. For them social and economic influences on health are very important and they are very much aware of the limitations of modern medicine which they consider needs demystifying so that people's understanding of health might be increased. Related to this is the idea that GPs require other attributes than just medical ones and need to be counsellors and educators.

10 marks

2. What groups do and how they do it

- It is self-evident that all health care is ineffective if it is inaccessible, if it is unacceptable and if it fails to relate to patient needs, which must therefore be identified in order to make optimum use of available resources. There are local differences but collectively the groups attempt to fill five major roles. First, the groups act as a planning tool by providing the primary health care team with information about patient needs, concerns and interests. Second, they act as a safety valve by providing an outlet for patient grumbles and complaints about the practice. Third, they allow the arrangement, as required, of health education lectures and discussion. Fourth, they provide a back-up service for the practice patients by organizing voluntary care in the community. Finally, they can attempt to act as the eyes and ears of the locality, feeding back information about needs to other parts of the health service. In pursuit of these aims, activities might include transport to the surgery, a prescription collecting service, modification of an appointment system, groups for alcoholics and slimmers, and pre-retirement classes.

25 marks

3. The benefits/costs

- Perhaps the most important question the groups will have to address themselves to is what difference will the existence of a patient participation group make to the individual patient on the list? The possibilities are many but they will not necessarily be measured purely in terms of longevity or morbidity. The quality of life is no less important, and self-care, patient compliance, contentment with the service and the relevance of the service are all important benefits that could result.
- Take up a lot of doctor time, especially initially, and may be difficult to judge just how representative of all patients some of the, usually self-selected, members are.

15 marks

Further reading

RCGP Occasional Paper No. 17: *Patient Participation in General Practice*

Q3   *What is terminal care? Discuss the role of the general practitioner. How should you respond if a patient you are treating asks about euthanasia?*

A3   **1. Preamble**

- The need for terminal care is probably easier to recognize than define. It has to do with the realization in doctor, family and patient that death is inevitable, even imminent, and that special attention is needed.
- The elements that may lead to recognition of the need for terminal care include:

    i.   Increasing pain.
    ii.   Decreasing mobility – even staying in bed.
    iii. Increasing anxiety in patient and/or carers.
    iv. Increase in intensity of other problems, e.g. breathlessness, bowel disturbance, depression.

20 marks

2. The role of the GP

It is wide-ranging but it has boundaries – other disciplines, nurses, social workers, night sitters may be in a position to offer better care.

- It must be negotiated with the patient and those who provide care on a day-to-day basis – family, friends, team members.
- It includes adequate pain relief.
- It includes adequate relief of other physical symptoms, e.g. breathlessness.
- It includes adequate explanation of what to expect to patient and family.
- It includes identifying the causes for concern and anxieties that patient and family have.
- It includes referral to other team members or consultant colleagues.
- It includes the provision of relief for those who do the caring, e.g. hospital care, temporary hospital or hospice admission as needed.
- It must include the development of a relationship of trust which allows the above to happen.

30 marks

3. Euthanasia

If a patient receiving terminal care 'asks about euthanasia', one should:

- Try to find out why the patient has put the question. 'What leads you to say that?' can be a useful response.
- Review the adequacy of the care one is providing in the light of the answers. Is the patient feeling a burden to others, is he in pain or distressed, is he depressed?
- Explain that the word euthanasia means 'easy death' and that the general practitioner will ensure that death will be easy in that adequate doses of all necessary drugs will be given to ensure that – even if life is shortened in the process.

- Explain that to give drugs in doses that are needed in order to kill directly is:
  i. Against the law.
  ii. Against the 'ethos' or ethical ideas of the medical profession, e.g. Hippocratic Oath.
  iii. Has an effect on the individual GP and his own views about his work. Explain one's own moral views.
  iv. A way of avoiding the real problems.
  v. Most important – with adequate communication between doctor–patient and carers it should be unnecessary.

40 marks

10 discretionary marks

This question tests, not only your understanding of the elements that constitute 'terminal care', but also your ideas about the boundaries between the role of the GP and other team members – including the role perhaps of a spiritual adviser. It also requires you to respond to a difficult problem in a caring humane way within the legal restraints that society imposes on doctors and the ethical–moral restraints that doctors impose on themselves.

The Orals

The tradition of oral examinations is a long and not altogether honourable one. Past candidates may have memories of orals that went wrong due to their own anxiety, misunderstandings with examiners, apparently irrelevant or unclear questions and, occasionally, frank personal animosity. Nevertheless, this is the only occasion on which candidates and examiners meet face-to-face, instead of as disembodied numbers on sheets of paper. The oral provides an unrivalled opportunity for the examiner to assess the performance of the candidate across a much broader range of attributes than any written paper could possibly achieve.

The aim, therefore, has been to train the examiners and arrange the orals in such a way that valuable features are conserved while unfair aspects are excluded as far as possible. Theoretically, an oral examination could be used to assess factual knowledge, patient management skills and attitudes to a wide variety of problems. However, it has become increasingly clear that the orals should concentrate on areas which cannot be adequately assessed in any other way. After all, bringing together over a hundred examiners and over a thousand candidates in Edinburgh or London for two half-hour vivas is an extraordinarily expensive exercise.

While it is evident that clinical medicine cannot be practised satisfactorily without a good deal of factual knowledge, this has already been tested in the MCQ and is not currently emphasized in the orals. Instead, the examiners concentrate on exploring the candidates' decision-making and problem-solving skills. As in the MEQ, the candidate will be expected to generate a range of options, which appear reasonable within the context of general practice, and to consider the advantages and disadvantages of each option. When finally pressed to make a decision, he or she will be expected to present a coherent argument to justify the chosen course of action. The advantage of this approach is that it prevents the examiner from judging the candidate solely on whether or not they both might reach the same final conclusion. It must be remembered that the examiners are real GPs and they will not be impressed by answers that are unlikely to be put into practice in real life.

Even more difficult is the assessment of attitudes. Indeed, some would claim that it is totally unjustifiable to consider attitudes in an examination, because beliefs and expressed attitudes are personal attributes entirely unrelated to professional practice and therefore no business of the College. However, a moment's reflection will demonstrate that it is often a doctor's attitude and behaviour, rather than factual knowledge or problem-solving skills, which dictate the quality of his or her practice. Thus attitudes are a valid area of concern, though this does not imply that there is an official 'College' attitude on every issue to which the candidate must conform. Rather, candidates must be aware of their own attitudes and those of others who may differ from them and show that they can understand the relevant implications. The examiners are not judging whether or not a candidate's attitudes coincide with their own, but whether the candidate is sensitive to those issues which may affect patients and colleagues profoundly.

Anxiety about these difficult areas of

assessment led the panel of examiners into undertaking an extensive study of the 'attributes' they would look for in a good candidate. Material generated by this study was subsequently arranged into seven 'areas of competence' which include accurate problem definition, skills in patient management, prevention, communication, organization, professional values and personal and professional growth. These have now been incorporated into the marking sheets completed by the examiners during each viva and this has helped to ensure wider and more consistent coverage of the whole range of topics concerned.

Marking

New examiners undergo an elaborate training programme which involves role-played and videotaped mock orals with feedback and this process continues into the examination itself. There will often be a third person present at the table in addition to the pair of examiners. He or she will either be a trainee examiner or another examiner whose role is to observe the oral and later comment on the other examiners' performance. A variant of this technique is to video a whole series of orals with an unobtrusive camera located behind the candidate, focused on the examiners. The examiners concerned are subsequently invited to study the tapes with an expert adviser and take note of aspects of their technique which require improvement.

Examiner pairs are changed frequently and great emphasis is placed on consistency and reliability of marking. Each day, examiners are required to watch and mark a videotaped oral as a calibration exercise and careful records are kept throughout the oral of topics covered and marks awarded at each stage.

Each examiner will have tried to make an assessment within the first 15–20 minutes as to whether the candidate seems likely to fail, pass comfortably or gain outstanding marks in this particular viva. He or she is then in a position either to raise the standard of questions in order to stretch a distinction candidate or revert to bread and butter issues if failure seems likely. Thus, paradoxically, the more demanding the viva becomes the more likely it is that the candidate

has done well and the easier it becomes, the higher the risk of failure. So, do not get flustered if your oral gets fiercer.

At the end of each oral, both examiners must commit themselves to record an overall mark before discussing the candidate with their partner and arriving at a final agreed mark.

Thus the 'hawks' and the 'doves' are made well aware of their tendencies and, indeed, may be required to defend their decisions in a 'quartet' discussion. This arises when the total marks of a candidate, including those from the written papers and both orals, place him or her marginally below the pass mark. In such cases both examiner pairs meet, with a senior examiner if necessary, in order to justify the marks awarded and consider the possibility of raising one or both oral marks in order to allow the candidate to pass. Strenuous attempts are made to ensure that the inherently valid technique of oral examinations becomes reliable as well.

Format

The two orals in the MRCGP examination are designed to explore performance from two rather different viewpoints. The first oral is based on the log diary, for which the candidate is required to complete a proforma detailing many aspects of practice organization and make a record of 50 consecutive patients he or she has seen and managed. The examiners use the information provided to explore the candidate's strengths and weaknesses *vis-à-vis* practice organization and patient management.

The second oral is designated as a problem-solving oral, in which the examiners present problems which they have encountered in their own practices and attempt to judge the adequacy of the response. Information may be provided verbally, in written form, as slides or colour photographs, as pathology, radiology or other reports, or in the form of an electrocardiographic tracing. Thus the skills of information gathering, hypothesis formation and testing, and patient management are assessed and this is the nearest point at which the examination approaches a true test of clinical skills.

Setting

About 80 per cent of all the candidates are invited to attend for the oral examinations. These are currently held in London, Edinburgh and Dublin. It is important to be aware that an invitation to the orals does not mean that the candidate has achieved a pass mark in the written papers, only that he or she is not so far below the pass mark as to have no chance of passing overall, no matter how good the performance in the orals. Thus, a candidate with good marks in the written papers may still pass after a couple of borderline orals, while the candidate with indifferent marks on the written papers, will ultimately fail if his or her oral marks are on the same borderline.

It is worth arriving a few minutes early for the examination so that you have time to compose yourself and enjoy a cup of coffee before the ordeal. Remember that the examiners are all in active general practice and usually actively involved in learning and teaching. A very high proportion are trainers, course organizers or members of academic departments of general practice. They are not out to intimidate you or threaten you, but they are skilled at searching out weak points and inconsistencies in your responses and it is most important that you get as much practice as possible beforehand in presenting your views and experience in a coherent and impressive manner.

By far the best way to gain experience in this respect is to practice mock vivas with the aid of friends, colleagues, teachers and examiners. If it is possible to audiotape or videotape these mock vivas then this will enable you to see for yourself where any potential difficulties may lie.

Remember to bring with you an aide memoire related to the 50 cases which you recorded in your log diary. Dress and appearance are a personal matter, but most candidates still seem to present their most conservative aspect on such occasions.

Each oral lasts about 25 minutes. A bell or gong is sounded at the end of time and you will be given your log diary and a sheet of paper to pass on to the second pair of examiners. This contains information about the topics covered in the first oral but you will not find any marks on it!

The log-diary oral

The log diary which you will have completed some weeks before the oral examination is illustrated on pp. 167–172. This has been in use for a long time now and may well be updated and modified within the next few years. It is important to note that the log diary itself is not marked as part of the examination. It is a tool which enables the examiners to place your experience within a given context, to enable you to evaluate the strengths, weaknesses and idiosyncracies of the practice in which you work and to provide 'pegs' on which to hang discussion about issues of practice management and organization. In addition, the 50 cases which you have recorded serve as useful starting points for discussion on clinical topics.

It is clearly not possible for the examiners to control the mix of cases which you choose to present but obvious 'plants' are usually studiously avoided. It is much better to provide a genuine list of consecutive cases and make sure that you have updated your aide memoire so that you can provide relevant information if required. There is really no excuse for failing to be adequately prepared for an oral examination focused on your own practice and your own patients! If you are not in active general practice in the UK then it is well worth undertaking some locum work, without payment if necessary, in order to have some fresh, live case material to which you can relate. It will also serve to remind you of the particular circumstances of NHS general practice.

Most examiners start by asking a couple of unmarkable questions about the practice in order to put the candidate at ease. The only topic of substance likely to arise from the first page relates to question 8, the obstetric commitment of the practice. This obviously provides a rich source of discussion about attitudes, as does the next question, on night visits. The pros and cons of appointment systems and special clinics within a practice also provide a lot of material.

If the candidate is a trainee he or she cannot, of course, be held responsible for the organization of the practice. Nevertheless, trainees should be prepared to assess their teaching practice critically and be aware of alternative ways of managing a practice. They should be familiar with the various roles of employed staff and have some knowledge of NHS regulations in respect of reimbursement payments. As future employers they should also be aware of their responsibilities, including the legal, financial, health and ethical aspects of managing staff. Experience suggests that the practice manager is usually the best source of information on this topic.

The selection, training and professional expertise of the other members of the primary health care team are very important and the examiners will have a keen appreciation of whether or not the candidate is likely to be able to work with them to provide a comprehensive service to the patients. If the practice boasts an impressive array of additional diagnostic equipment then that is fine, but you, as the candidate, must be aware of the correct application and maintenance of the equipment as well as its clinical usage. Remember that a little knowledge may be a dangerous thing! Access to diagnostic facilities is again probably outside the trainee's, and often the principal's, control, but you may be asked how you might respond if, for instance, open access to contrast radiological studies was suddenly withdrawn at your local hospital. You would also be expected to have a rough idea of the relative costs of some common investigations.

On page 3 of the log diary you are invited to draw attention to any special features of the practice which you may wish to emphasize. This might include a note about the geographical area in which the practice is situated, the age–sex and social class distribution of the patient population and any special registers or research interests which the practice may have. You should be prepared to answer questions about the likely influence of these factors on the way the practice functions and to contrast this with other types of practice in different localities. Similarly you should have an idea of how the practice workload (page 4) compares with local and national averages and be prepared to speculate on why this may be.

Although the first part of the log diary provides a rich source of discussion, it is unlikely that the examiners will spend more than 10 minutes on this area. They are always keen to get on to your cases and to see how you handle your own patients in the surgery and at home. This is where your aide memoire comes in. A few days before the oral it is wise to review your cases again, asking yourself a series of questions about your diagnosis and management, whether there were alternative ways in which you might have dealt with the situation and whether, in retrospect, you would have handled things differently. A run-through with your trainer or a colleague can be very helpful in this respect.

Nevertheless, you must remember that the examiners are not bound to stick with your cases and are quite likely to lead you into other areas if the opportunity arises. The whole essence of an oral examination is the unparalleled flexibility it provides for the examiners to explore your knowledge, skills and attitudes in any area which seems appropriate at the time.

PRACTICE LOG
Analysis of Work Load and Practice Organization

NAME: ...... **A. Trainee** ....

Examination
number: **0123** ......

ADDRESS: ...... **'Meadowcroft', Highfield Road, Airportville, Sussex** ....

The following analysis will assist the Panel of Examiners to assess you in your examination performance.

The audit will not in itself attract any marks but will help the examiners to enquire into your knowledge of practice organization and discuss with you the patients you have seen recently.

Please complete pages 1, 2, 3 and 4 and on pages 5 and 6 record details of 50 consecutive patients seen.

1. *Practice List Size*

   10 694

2. *Your Status in the Practice –*

   Principal [ ]   Assistant [ ]   Trainee [x]

3. *Length of Experience in General Practice*   **1 year**

4. *Number of Years in Post*   **1 year**

5. *Type of Practice*

   Rural [ ]   Urban [x]   Mixed [ ]   Dispensing [ ]   Teaching [x]

6. *Type of Premises*

   Converted [**2 x**]   Purpose Built [ ]   Health Centre [ ]

7. *Total Number of Doctors in the Practice* (Providing General Medical Services)

   Full-time partners   **4**

   Part-time partners   **2**

   Assistants   **–**

   Trainee Assistants   **2**

8. *Obstetric Commitment of the Practice*

    Number of confinements in complete care

    | 38 |

    Number of confinements in shared care

    | 11 |

    (These figures should refer to a recent quarter for which figures are available)

9. *Total number of night visits (11 p.m. – 7 a.m.) made by the candidate during the most recent complete month*

    | 1 |

10. *Appointments System*   YES ~~NO~~   FULL ~~PARTIAL~~

11. *Special Sessions: Specify*
    e.g. Antenatal Clinic
          Immunization
          Cytology

    Antenatal Clinic × 2
    Immunization Clinic × 2
    Well Man Clinic
    Well Woman Clinic
    Well Baby Clinic

12. *Staff Employed: Specify*

    Practice Manager (full-time)
    Secretary (part time)
    Receptionists/Clerks (part time) × 16
    Practice Nurses (part time) × 3

13. *Staff Attached: Specify*

    District Nurses SRN × 2
    District Nurse SEN
    District Auxiliary
    Health Visitors × 3
    Community Psychiatric Nurse

14. *Additional Diagnostic Equipment*
    e.g. ECG, Peak Flow Meter

    ECG
    Peak Flow Meters

15. *Diagnostic Facilities to which open or direct access is available: Specify*

    All Radiology
    All Pathology
    Physiotherapy
    Occupational Therapy

16. *Post held outwith the Practice, e.g. Hospital Sessions*

Associate Regional Adviser   –   3 sessions

2 × Course Organizers   –   2 sessions each

Clinical Assistantships in Mental Subnormality   –   5 sessions

17. *Any special Characteristics of your Practice to which you wish to draw attention, e.g. Teaching, Geographical Features, Social Features:*

The practice is situated close to a major airport and thriving industrial estate so incomes are relatively high and unemployment low. Patients are mostly social class 3 and 4 and about 12 per cent are immigrants from the Indian subcontinent. All of the partners are involved in educational pursuits, either within the practice or outside.

TOTAL PRACTICE WORK LOAD OVER ONE WEEK

1. *No. of patients seen by all doctors –*

	M	Tu	W	Th	F	Sat
Consulting a.m.	61	57	69	51	59	–
Consulting p.m.	44	38	–	37	45	–
Other surgeries or special clinics	21	14	6	16	–	–
New home visits	16	11	11	5	7	
Repeat home visits			Not differentiated			

2. *No. of patients seen by the Candidate –*

	M	Tu	W	Th	F	Sat
Consulting a.m.	13	12	14	12	13	–
Consulting p.m.	12	14	–	–	13	–
Other surgeries or special clinics	7	–	6	–	–	–
New home visits	2	2	2	1	1	–
Repeat home visits	1	0	1	0	0	–

List consecutively 50 patients seen during the week of the audit, *in the consulting room and on home visits* (excluding special clinics).

As the examiners will wish to explore particular cases it will be in your own interest to bring an aide memoire with you.

V = Visit
S = Surgery

Case no.	Date	Patient's name or initials	Age	Sex	Main reasons for contact	V	S
1	22/7	Mr G.G.	43	M	Itchy eyes, headaches		x
2		Mr A.W.	57	M	Renal colic, 'flu		x
3		Mrs G.W.	53	F	Chronic low back pain		x
4		Mr G.L.	82	M	AF, CCF, skin rash		x
5		Mr P.L.	42	M	Blocked ears, anxiety		x
6		Mrs R.C.	71	F	For vaginal repair		x
7		Mr M.C.	54	M	Asthma		x
8		Mr G.C.	16	M	Hay fever		x
9		Mr F.H.	65	M	Hypertension		x
10		Miss P.H.	64	F	Injured toe + deafness		x
11		Mr M.S.	58	M	Piles		x
12		Mrs P.K.	32	F	Ex-laparoscopy, RIF pain		x
13		Mr A.M.	5	M	URTI, MSU		x
14		Mrs D.M.	34	F	Hay fever		x
15		Mr B.M.	8	M	Scarletina	x	
16		Mrs R.C.	85	F	OA, mild CCF	x	
17		Miss V.L.	19	F	Oral contraception mild vaginismus		x
18		Mrs G.F.	54	F	Hypertension, angina		x
19		Mrs J.B.	61	F	Hip replacement		x
20		Miss J.L.	6	F	'Hyperactive'		x
21		Mrs B.L.	41	F	Migraine		x
22		Miss A.P.	18	F	Acne		x
23		Mr J.G.	12	M	Pharyngitis		x
24		Mr P.S.	42	M	Ankylosing spondylitis		x
25		Mrs M.C.	37	F	Oral contraception		x

Case no.	Date	Patient's name or initials	Age	Sex	Main reasons for contact	V	S
26	22/7	Mr F.B.	45	M	Lumbago and sciatica		x
27		Mr T.G.	59	M	Diabetes		x
28		Miss H.C.	12	F	Hay fever		x
29		Mr G.W.	71	M	Psoriasis, cancer of prostate		x
30		Mr K.P.	36	M	Schizophrenia		x
31	23/7	Mr F.C.	66	M	Terminal malignancy	x	
32		Mr W.F.	3	M	Otitis media		x
33		Mrs J.K.	28	F	? allergy to eye make-up		x
34		Mrs J.W.	52	F	Bunions and varicose veins		x
35		Mr A.P.	38	M	Epilepsy		x
36		Mrs J.B.	52	F	Thyrotoxicosis		x
37		Mr R.B.	44	M	Recurrent knee pain		x
38		Mrs J.K.	50	F	Chronic anxiety		x
39		Mr S.D.	26	M	Haemophilia		x
40		Miss M.P.	4	F	URTI, cough		x
41		Mr A.W.	53	M	Hypertension		x
42		Miss H.G.	18	F	Oral contraception + *Candida*		x
43		Mrs R.N.	36	F	Cervical smear		x
44		Mrs A.B.	72	F	OA hips and knees		x
45		Mr D.S.	4	M	URTI, earache		x
46		Mr A.N.	16	M	Eczema and asthma		x
47		Mr J.G.	68	M	Chronic bronchitis		x
48		Miss B.B.	7/12	F	Feeding and sleeping problems		x
49		Mrs G.H.	44	F	Pelvic inflammatory disease	x	
50		Mrs P.J.	88	F	Mild dementia, mild CCF	x	

The problem-solving oral

The second oral takes place on the examiner's ground rather than your own. Nevertheless, an understanding of the type and range of answers expected will help you to tune-in to what the examiners expect and perform well. The nearest equivalent part of the examination to the second oral is the MEQ and many of the same principles apply. However, unlike the MEQ, the examiner is able to manipulate his cases as he goes along, following highways and byways if they look promising and even expand on his colleague's cases when the opportunity presents. Thus no two orals will ever be quite the same, even if the cases presented are identical, and the responses of the candidate may profoundly alter the course which the oral takes.

Think before you speak or your answer may trigger off a series of questions which expose an area of ignorance or incompetence. It does no harm to clarify a question if you are genuinely unclear as to what the examiner is getting at, but beware of irritating mannerisms such as always repeating the question to yourself. Some candidates can be a pleasure to examine, discussion flows freely and a lot of ground is covered. Other candidates are so slow, hesitant or obtuse that few topics are completed and the examiners may find it difficult to know what level of mark to give.

Some examples of the type of question which may be asked, and the range of answers expected are provided below. You will see that although they are predominantly based on case material, there are also some which invite you to speculate on more general issues, such as may crop up in the PTQ.

Specimen oral questions

A   Long cases

A1 Mr X, aged 38 years, has a history of recurrent attacks of lethargy which, in the past, have been diagnosed as anxiety/depression and which apparently have been successfully treated. He has seen your partner only 3 days ago who made

this diagnosis because of lethargy over the preceding 4 weeks. Mr X asks to be referred to a specialist.

Analysis (by examinee)
- The diagnosis has not been successfully negotiated with the patient.
- The management already offered has not been acceptable.
- Reluctance to refer at this stage.
- Concern about the partner–patient relationship.

Questions (by examiner)
- *Are there any other possible diagnoses?*
- *How would you manage this patient?*
- *Would you say anything to your partner?*

Response (by examinee)
- Lethargy can be a symptom of virtually any physical or psychological disorder. It is necessary to allow the patient to tell his story again including his own ideas, concerns and expectations.
- Clinical examination is necessary for assessment and reassurance paying particular attention to appetite, weight, urinalysis. The patient must feel that he is being taken seriously. There may be a need to investigate this patient depending on assessment results from history and examination. A blood test may be negotiated as a satisfactory alternative to a referral. Referral is difficult when you feel you should attempt management yourself. However, the patient should learn that the outcome will be satisfactory in a few weeks and, if it isn't, a referral will then take place.
- These sort of patients make an ideal case to discuss at practice meetings. What would other partners do in this situation?
- What is the practice attitude to personal care? Should the original doctor have seen this patient in the first place or should the patient have a right to consult elsewhere?

A2 Your receptionist tells you shortly after you arrive at 8.45 a.m. on a Monday morning that a patient is asking to speak to you urgently; although you are not on call for the practice, there is no other doctor around. *On speaking to the patient (a 35-year-old male executive) you learn that he has been in sudden severe pain (left-sided colicky abdominal pain radiating to the scotum) and that he rang the duty doctor at 8 a.m. and was told to ring again after 8.30 a.m. when the surgery opened.*

Analysis (by examinee)
- This sounds like ureteric colic.
- This pain must be stopped at once (by me or the doctor on call).
- Need to review the deputizing arrangements.

Questions (by examiner)
- **What is the likely diagnosis?**
- **What do you say to the patient and what immediate steps would you take?**
- **How would you establish the diagnosis?**
- **How would you manage the patient?**
- **What is the likely prognosis and outcome?**

Response (by examinee)
- Ureteric colic.
- Patient is told a doctor will come at once. Possibly doctor on call can see the patient on his way in if he is contactable. If not I will go.
- Immediate priority is pain relief; parenteral morphine with an antiemetic can be given intravenously or intramuscularly. Three fundamental questions exist (after relief of severe pain):

  > Is this urolithiasis?
  > Are there any underlying causes?
  > Are there any complications?

  The second and third questions could wait until after morning surgery as could substantiation of the first.
- Diagnosis established by history and investigations on the stone (if one is passed), the urine and the blood.
- Patient advised to drink plenty of fluids and take adequate analgesics. Patient told to send for help if pain relief not adequate. Enlist help of District Nursing Service. Admit to hospital if pain relief not adequate, anuria develops or pain lasts longer than 24–48 hours.

- Recurrence is usual. Specialist help is needed including radiological investigation and consideration for surgery.

B   Short cases

B1 *You receive at 4 p.m. a telephone call from Mrs Y. You remember treating her 6-year-old son with amoxycillin 3 weeks ago because he had otitis media. Mrs Y has just 'cleaned out' the boy's ear because of wax and now he has earache. She can't bring hom down to the surgery because she has just had an operation and Mr Y has gone to work in his car.*

Analysis (by examinee)
- A home visit should not be necessary.
- The pain is probably traumatic in origin.

Questions (by examiner)
- **What do you say to the mother?**
- **How would you manage the situation?**

Response (by examinee)
- Explain that the likely cause is trauma. Advise analgesia and to ring back if pain does not disappear within 30 minutes.
- Review the boy at the surgery at the earliest convenient opportunity.

B2 *A routine blood test carried out by the Blood Transfusion Service reveals that a 45-year-old male patient is HIV positive. He consults you and asks why he has been turned down.*

Assessment (by examinee)
- Need to be frank.
- Need for sensitivity.
- What does the patient suspect already?

Questions (by the examiner)
- **What would you do?**

Response (by examinee)
- Find out what the patient suspects already. Reflect the patient's question 'what have you been telling yourself about the situation?'.
- If the patient is homosexual or a drug addict, lifestyle changes will be needed (steady partners, non-penetrating sex). Need to consult one of the advisory services, e.g. Terence Higgins Trust.

- Patient should not have children. Explain incubation period is at least 2 years. Need to be optimistic about outlook and to establish relationship of trust.

C   Non-clinical questions

C1   The White Paper on the Primary Care Services

- *What is it?*
- *What did it recommend?*
- *What do you think about it?*
- *What do the RCGP and the BMA think about it?*

C2   The Primary Health Care Team

- *What will the GP be doing at turn of the century?*
- *What will the nurse be doing at the turn of the century?*

C3   The cost of the Health Service

- *How do we compare with other countries?*
- *Relative costs of primary and secondary services.*
- *Precribing costs.*

D   Bread and butter cases

D1   A patient makes an urgent appointment because she has forgotten her contraceptive pill.

- *What do you say?*
- *What do you do?*

D2   A 46-year-old lady tells you that she will not keep you long and that she would like a prescription for vitamin pills.

- *Why might she have come to see you when she could buy them?*
- *How would you manage this situation?*

D3   A 24-year-old lady presents with a chronic recurrent red eye.

The diagnosis is allergic conjunctivitis.

- *What treatment options exist?*
- *In what circumstances would you prescribe local steroids?*

Mock Orals

The log diary is designed to evaluate candidates' knowledge, skills and attitudes in relation to their own patients, while the problem-solving oral is based on the examiner's cases and issues.

The candidate should be expected to know enough about other types of practice, and their problems and difficulties, to be able to compare and contrast experience with that of colleagues in other parts of the UK and, to a lesser extent, other parts of the world.

It should be remembered that medical knowledge has been extensively tested in the written papers, especially the MCQs, so do not spend too much time and effort in asking straightforward factual questions.

The great advantage of oral examinations is their flexibility. You are in a position, therefore, to assess the candidate's decision-making and problem-solving skills in depth and also to explore attitudes towards patients colleagues.

It is most important that you do not assess the candidate simply on the basis of whether or not he or she did what you would have done in a similar situation. The way to avoid this is to ask him or her to consider the options at any given point and what the advantages and disadvantages of any course of action might be.

When a preferred course of action is chosen, challenge it so it can be justified in a rational and coherent manner.

The exploration of attitudes is even more difficult but probably even more vital. Again, it is most important to avoid judging simply on the basis that views coincide with yours.

To avoid this trap, try to explore whether or not he or she appreciates that there are valid alternative attitudes held by colleagues and encourage exploration of the implications of these varying attitudes.

When discussing clinical cases or practice organization, it is worth checking that actual behaviour is consistent with the attitudes expressed.

A fierce expression of the value of an intensely personal style of practice would hardly be consistent with practice in a group which makes no provision for continuity of care and uses a deputizing service every night and weekend.

You should keep a record of all the topics covered in the vivas and assign marks to each topic on a 10-point scale, using 5 as the borderline. Thus an excellent response on a particular topic might rate 8–10, while an adequate response might merit a 6, and a good response 7. Conversely, a barely adequate series of answers might score 4 and a totally inadequate response 3 or less.

Averaging out the topic marks at the end of the viva will give you an approximate overall score, but you will probably want to make some allowance for the relative importance of the various topics covered.

If the candidate is doing well it is important to increase the difficulty and depth of the questions as you go along so you give a fair chance of obtaining distinction level marks.

If he is doing badly, you may need to resort to bread and butter issues and straightforward management situations so you will feel justified in failing him if he does not come up to scratch.

The log-diary oral (25–30 minutes)

You should spend a few minutes before the candidate comes in looking at the log diary, picking out any points which stand out, and looking through the cases so you can plan your strategy.

The problem-solving oral (25–30 minutes)

In the real examination, the candidate would have a break of not more than 5 minutes between the two orals and would go to a different pair of examiners carrying a note of the topics covered in the first oral to avoid duplication.

Preparation for this second oral places considerable responsibility on the examiner, who must choose the issues and cases carefully, work out the range of answers which he thinks the candidate may produce, and decide what is really being looked for in each instance. In addition, be flexible and be prepared to deviate if an important new topic arises and seems worthwhile pursuing.

Either use your own cases and problems as a basis for the oral or use the sample cases that follow.

Specimens

Case 1

A 4-year-old boy is brought along by his mother. She says that he had earache overnight, but he appears bright and chirpy. How would you manage this situation?

Answers expected
- Good general assessment, approach to child.
- Appearance of drum (you may be given a colour picture or slide) – interpretation.
- Management options – antibiotics or not? (Quote recent papers if possible)
- Explanation to mother.
- Possible complications.
- Follow-up – why and when?

Supplementary questions
What is meant by the term 'glue ear'?
How can it be prevented?
What are the management options?

Answers expected
- Definition, natural history.
- Assessment, emphasis on deafness and effects on learning.
- Value of nasal drops, oral decongestants, antihistamines.
- Indications for referral.
- Advice to parents re grommets, swimming etc.

Case 2

What were the main findings of the recent MRC Hypertension Study? What implications does it have for general practice?

Answers expected
- Study looked at mild–moderate hypertension in general practice using funded nurses.
- Treatment with bendrofluazide or propranolol.
- No reduction of overall mortality.
- Some reduction in stroke (but 850 patient-years' treatment necessary to prevent one stroke).
- No reduction in mortality from coronary heart disease.

- Appreciable incidence of side-effects, e.g. lassitude, impotence, mild diabetes.
- Most important step is to stop smoking!

Supplementary question
How might you organize your practice to detect and care for patients with hypertension?

Answers expected
- Discussion of case-finding *vs* screening. Need for follow-up, recall, repeat prescribing systems.
- Importance of developing practice policies.

Case 3

You have a patient of 64 with a very painful arthritic hip. There is a 2-year waiting list for hip replacement locally. What can you do to help?

Answers expected
- General measures, e.g. weight loss, walking stick, analgesics.
- Personal approach to consultant.
- Refer elsewhere with shorter waiting list (College of Health has information).
- Discuss possibility of private operation – if insured or wealthy (cost £3000–£5000).
- Local or national medico-political action, e.g. District Management team, District Health Authority, MP, British Medical Association etc.

Case 4

A middle-aged lady asks for your help with her husband who is drinking too much. How would you approach this problem?
What help can you offer?

Answers expected
- Exploration of the problem – what effects is it having on family, employment etc?
- Sympathetic understanding and support.
- Offer help if husband can be persuaded to attend voluntarily.
- Consider personal invitation to attend, possibly for general check-up, blood pressure etc.

- If unsuccessful, advise with reference to voluntary agencies or other sources of help.
- Stress continuing availability.

Supplementary question
How would you help her husband if he approached you personally?

Answers expected
- Assessment of physical, psychological, social state.
- Investigations, e.g. γ-glutamyl transpeptidase, mean corpuscular volume, liver function tests.
- Sympathetic support and advice, regular follow-up.
- Possible involvement of Community Psychiatric Nurse, Alcoholics Anonymous etc.
- Referral to psychiatrist or alcoholic unit.

Case 5

A man of 38 has a history of recurrent attacks of lethargy which, in the past, have been diagnosed as anxiety/depression and apparently treated successfully. He was seen by your partner 3 days ago and started on antidepressants. He asks to be referred to a specialist. What may be behind this request? How could you manage the problem?

Answers expected
- Clearly, your partner has not been successful in negotiating the diagnosis with the patient.
- Therefore, the treatment offered is not acceptable at this point.
- You should be concerned about the relationship between your partner and the patient. (Point for discussion about personal lists.)
- Referral may not be appropriate.
- Reconsider diagnosis – may be physical, psychological or social causes for lethargy.
- Explore patient's ideas, concerns, expectations.
- Need for appropriate history, examination and, if necessary, investigation.
- Explain findings and negotiate management with patient.

- Keep option of referral open.
- Communicate with partner. Possibly discuss case at practice meeting, tutorial etc.

Case 6

You arrive at work at 8.45 a.m. on a Monday morning ready to start a large, booked surgery. The receptionist tells you that a patient is on the phone who wishes to speak to you urgently.

He is a 35-year-old male executive who tells you that he has had severe pain for the past hour. It is localized in the left loin and the left side of the abdomen and radiates to the groin. He rang the Duty Doctor, who works in a neighbouring practice, at 8 a.m. and was told to ring again after 8.30 a.m. when the surgery opened.

What problems does this situation present? How would you handle them?

Answers expected
- Immediate priority is diagnosis and pain relief – ? ureteric colic – visit, administer appropriate analgesic.
- Receptionist will have to explain situation to patients waiting – either wait, rebook or see another doctor if available.
- Revisit after surgery for review, explanation and consideration of further investigation – stone, urine, blood tests, referral etc.
- Advise plenty of fluids, provide adequate analgesia, stress availability, ? involve district nurse or psychiatric nurse.
- May need hospital admission if pain relief not adequate, anuria develops or pain persists longer than 24–48 hours.
- Need to review deputizing arrangements. Discuss with colleague on call.

Case 7

A routine test carried out by the Blood Transfusion Service reveals that a 45-year-old male patient is HIV positive. He consults you and aks why he has been turned down as a donor.

How would you reply? What can you do to help him?

Answers expected
- The doctor must be honest and frank with the patient, while remaining sensitive to the implications of the finding.
- Explore the patient's suspicions and fears.
- Explain the medical facts.
- Discuss the patient's lifestyle – likely to be homosexual or drug addict. Risk of infecting others sexually.
- Advise him to consult one of the advisory services, e.g. Terence Higgins Trust.
- Offer continuing advice, support and follow-up. Try to establish a relationship of trust.

Cast 8

What is the Third National Morbidity Survey? What information does it provide?

Answers expected
- A joint research exercise by the RCGP, OPCS and DHSS undertaken in 1980–81 and published in 1986. (Previous surveys 1955–56 and 1970–71.)
- About 150 GPs from 50 practices from all over the country took part, keeping a record of all consultations for a year.
- Results provided information on:
  Annual consultation rate per patient (3.4).
  Percentage of patients consulting per annum (71 per cent).
  Main reasons for consultation – major categories were respiratory disorders, 'symptoms', preventive measures etc.

Supplementary questions
There is a large scope for discussion about the variability of consultation rates between doctors, practices, parts of the country and internationally. In addition, comparison may be made with findings from other sources.

Case 9

What is the average number of prescriptions written per person per annum? How much do they cost? What are your views on this?

Answers expected
- In 1986, there were seven scripts written

for each person in the UK, 75 per cent are free.

- This implies that probably half are 'repeat prescriptions' issued without direct contact.
- Each GP costs the NHS well over £50 000 per year by his prescribing. There is huge variability in volume and costs between GPs – discuss information sources.
- Discuss ways of reducing costs, e.g. limited list, generic prescribing – pros and cons, discussion groups (quote evidence if possible).
- Britain is, in fact, well down the league when it comes to prescribing costs.

In questions like this, the examiners are not looking for 'pat' answers. They expect intelligent discussion, awareness of the issues and evidence of having given thought to the problems involved.

Case 10

What is your practice policy in relation to influenza immunization? How do you or might you organize the practice to provide this service?

Answers expected
- Contentious area – evidence of efficacy is limited and cost–benefit doubtful – discuss reasons for this.
- Nevertheless, it is recommended by DHSS for high-risk groups, and it may be profitable for the practice.
- Organization involves using the practice age–sex and disease register to call for patients, plus opportunistic immunization.
- Vaccine may be purchased directly from manufacturer or pharmacist and scripts written on EC 10 – most profitable arrangement!

Other areas of current interest which might well come up in the oral examinations include:
- The White Paper and the response of the RCGP and BMA.
- The 'Good Practice Allowance'.
- Standard-setting and medical audit.
- The future of the Primary Health Care Team – after Cumberledge.
- The future of the NHS.
- Prevention and screening.
- Demographic changes – how to cope with an increasingly elderly population.

Some Basic Facts and Figures

There are many data and statistics about general practice, its activities and its relationship with others. They are usually presented in a dull manner and difficult to understand.

However, it is important to have a grasp of facts and figures on the NHS and general practice to deal with questions and expand on answers in all parts of the examination.

It is helpful in the oral examination to relate your own log diary to the experience of other practices. It is helpful to refer to data in dealing with PTQs, with some MCQs and MEQs and, of course, it is up to you to introduce them in your free-ranging oral.

Sources of data

You should know the sources of data on general practice and the NHS if asked.

- *Health and Personal Social Services Statistics for England* is an annual publication of the DHSS and contains all basic data on the NHS.
- *Social Trends* is an annual by the Central Statistical Office with facts on social matters such as households and families, education, employment, income and wealth, health, housing, leisure and others.
- The *Morbidity Surveys* carried out by the College, the DHSS and the Office of Population Censuses and Surveys is the best source of morbidity in general practice; the latest, for 1981–2, was published in 1986.
- *NHS Data Book* is a digest of these and other sources (by J. Fry, D. Brooks and I.

McColl, published by MTP, Lancaster, 1984).
- *Medical Annual*, edited by D. J. P. Gray, published by Wright, Bristol, has some data in it.

Population and vital statistics

The population of the UK has been little changed since 1975 and with a fertility rate of only 1.75 (that is 1.75 children to a man and wife) the population will fall, but immigration may keep it stable.

UK population (in 1985) – 56.5 million
      over 65s   17%
      under 15s 18%

Annual birth rate – 12–13 per 1000 population
    per GP: 24–26 births

Annual death rate – 11–12 per 1000 population
    per GP: 22–24 deaths

The following provides a guide to our better health and standards of care.

Life expectancy (at birth)
    Males   72 years
    Females 78 years

Perinatal mortality rate – 10 per 1000 births

Maternal mortality rate – 0.08 per 1000 births

Cost of the NHS

It is necessary to note that the NHS is one of the largest government spenders financed largely (88 per cent) from central government funding or taxes.

In 1985 in the UK	
NHS costs were	£17 500 million
Personal social	
services costs were	£ 3 400 million
	£20 900 million
Costs per person for 1985	£370
Costs per GP	£600 000

The distribution of NHS costs	
Hospitals	63%
GPs	6%
GP prescribing	10%
	16%
Other	21%
	100%

Medical manpower in NHS (1985)

GPs	32 250
Hospitals	
Consultants	17 000
Junior hospital doctors	26 500
	43 500

Note 9500 GPs work in the hospitals as hospital practitioners (1000) and as clinical assistants (8500).

Of the 32 250 GPs in UK in 1985 there were	
Principals	30 000
Assistants	250
Trainees	2 000

GP list size

With a population of 56.5 million and 30 000 principals, the average list size was 1975 per GP. It was estimated to be:

England and Wales – 2000 per GP
N. Ireland   – 1950 per GP
Scotland   – 1700 per GP

Note in 1950 the average list size was 2500 patients and by 2000 it will be down to 1700.

Practice Units

The mean partnership size of a general practice now is between three and four GPs.

The percentage of GPs who work in the different size units are as follows:

Practice partnership size	*Percentage in*	
	1984	*1950*
×1 (solo) GP	12	43
×2 GPs	16	33
×3 GPs	22	15
×4 GPs	18	6
×5 or more	32	3

Note the great change from 1950 and the increase in large practice units.

Work in general practice – a profile

From the Third National Morbidity Survey and other sources the work profile is as follows:

Per year	
Annual patient consulting rate (patients who are seen by GP)	71%
Annual consultation rate (consultations per person) Surgery 3.0 Home visits 0.4	3.4
Per week Consultations Home visits	130 11 ── 141
Per day (5 day week) Consultations (13 per session) Home visits	26 2 ── 28
Night visits (11 p.m.–7 a.m.) 1 every 2 weeks	
Time per consultation (surgery) 5–10 minutes	

Prescribing

Between 60 and 70 per cent consultations include a prescription and there are also many 'repeat' prescriptions or prescriptions for 'unseen' patients.

For 1984	
Number of prescriptions per person per year	6.93
Average cost per prescription	£4.40
Cost of all prescriptions per person £30.50	
Prescribing costs per GP	£60 000

Note annual consultation is 3.4 and prescription rate is 6.93 – this suggests one-half of all prescriptions are for repeats etc. In 1984 the net income per GP was £24 000 and his prescribing costs were £60 000.

GP–hospital interface

About 1 in 10 of GP consultations involves referral to a hospital specialist.
But for the population as a whole in 1984:

Admitted to hospital	13%
Outpatients (new attenders)	18%
Accident – emergency (new attenders)	22%

It is likely that about 1 in 3 of the population is treated at hospital each year.

Costs of hospital care

In 1984 the costs for hospital care were as follows:

In-patient per week	
Teaching hospitals	
London	£845
Outside London	£725
Non-teaching hospitals	
Acute	£585
Maternity	£687
Geriatric	£263
Mental illness	£255
Out-patient attendance	£30

Suggestions

It is strongly recommended that examina tion candidates study, understand an memorize these data, that they try and relat it to their own training practices, and tha they study themselves some of the source of data to which they can refer as and whe appropriate.

Work Plan

The stated aim of the MRCGP examination is to test competence. It is not particularly difficult nor is it designed to fail or pass a certain fixed proportion of candidates. However, it is a demanding test of general practice knowledge and skills and is unlikely to be passed without careful preparation and a sound factual base. Do not underestimate the work involved; even the most confident can fail if they sit the examination without having refreshed and consolidated their knowledge and experience.

Everyone has his or her own preferred way of preparing for examinations, tried and tested through the undergraduate years. Our suggestions are pragmatic and have been found helpful by previous candidates.

The time to start preparing is 6 months or more before the written examination:

- Read the recommended journals (*Journal of the RCGP, Update*, the *British Medical Journal, Pulse* or other weekly journal, *Medeconomics*) regularly to provide a broad base of current knowledge and thought and make notes of any interesting points.
- Do general reading – recent textbooks of relevance to general practice.
- Attend local postgraduate and training meetings with GP topics. Take every opportunity to discuss and debate, with colleagues, all aspects of general practice.
- Pretend an examiner is constantly looking over your shoulder. Question your own attitudes and methods of working. Critically analyse each prescription, investigation, examination and referral that you issue or initiate. Hopefully you will

recognize and change your own questionable habits before they become exposed to others.
- Be aware of the regulations governing your everyday work. Carefully read the advice given in the book of Death Certificates, on a cremation form, in *Fitness to Drive*, on Med 3 and Med 5, National Insurance Certificates, in the *Red Book*, on the green 'abortion form' and so on. Do you know the criteria for sectioning a patient under the 1983 Mental Health Act?
- Three months before the written papers, plan and commence your individual revision programme. Two or three hours per night for four nights a week should be ample and rotating the subjects covered will avoid staleness. Plan to finish this programme a few days before the examination to allow everything to 'settle' in your mind.
- If possible, attend a short course or study day on the nuts and bolts of the examination. If you have time then consider going on an intensive or extended course as the opportunities for argument and debate with other candidates are valuable.
- Answer past or mock papers and even write a few essays. If you can find a friend to study with this can be of enormous help.
- After the written papers try to get together with other candidates or someone with experience of the examination (your trainer?) for discussion and mock oralling. The 'examiners' must be prepared to give honest feedback. Audio- or even videotaping of the vivas allows later critical self-analysis of technique.

Books and Journals

Medical journals

Although it is difficult sometimes to avoid feeling overwhelmed by the sheer volume of free literature that comes our way, selective reading of five or six of the journals most likely to contain information relevant to the examination is essential. The variety stimulates and even articles on the same subject can have slightly different information presented in very different ways.

While it is helpful for all of us to regularly read journals, from the examination point of view those of 6 months to a year before a particular examination are likely to be most valuable. Our personal recommendations are:

1. *Journal of the RCGP*
   Read the editorials and the 'News and Views' section. College reports and occasional papers are also well worth reading.
2. *British Medical Journal*
   Read the leading articles and the general practice section.
3. *Update*
   Use as a source of up-to-date revision material. Will be mostly relevant although omit too hospital orientated articles that may be in 'From the Postgraduate Centres'.
4. *Drug and Therapeutics Bulletin*
   Most authoritative and useful therapeutics information.
5. A weekly medical newspaper (*Pulse* or *General Practitioner*). Read to keep up with 'hot' medico-political issues.
6. *Medeconomics*
   Worth reading for information on practice organization and finance.

If you have the time, quickly flick through every journal that comes your way. Any one of them may contain the odd article covering an examination relevant topic in an interesting and useful way. Articles which catch your eye can be torn out and perused at leisure. Make short summary notes of any papers that interest you.

Books

There are now so many books relevant to general practice that it is impossible to mention them all. Most doctors will have their own preferences for reference books on specialist clinical subjects and will have acquired their own library of general practice books. We are therefore restricting our recommended book list to the essential minimum for day-to-day examination revision.

Clearly critical reading of other books, particularly on the consultation, team work and sociological aspects of practice, is highly desirable and the use of appropriate specialist texts is essential for revision of ophthalmology, dermatology etc.

1. *British National Formulary*
   Know this backwards. Contains a lot of medical as well as therapeutics information
2. An up-to-date general practice textbook.
   Use one of the general practice textbooks, e.g. *Management in General Practice*, by P. Pritchard, K. Low and M. Whalen, Oxford University Press, Oxford, 1984.

3. *Common Diseases* by J. Fry, Kluwer Academic Publishers, Norwell, MA, USA, 1983. A very easy book to revise from. Strengths are the simple and clear presentations and the truly practice-based perspective that it provides.
4. *Present State and Future Needs in General Practice,* by J. Fry, Kluwer Academic Publishers, Norwell, MA, USA, 1983.
   A quick read providing background facts and figures on general practice in Britain.
5. *Running a Practice: A Manual of Practice Management,* 3rd edn, by R. V. Jones, K. J. Bolden, D. J. Gray and M. S. Hall, Methuen, London, 1985.
   Deals with practice management and organization including the 'team'.
6. *Emergencies in General Practice,* 2nd edn, by A. J. Moulds, P. B. Martin and T. A. Bouchier-Hayes, Kluwer Academic Publishers, Norwell, MA, USA, 1986.
   A good book for the orals.

As part of the basic preparation it is also worth reading:

1. *Towards Earlier Diagnosis: A Guide to Primary Care,* 5th edn, by K. Hodgkin, Churchill Livingstone, Edinburgh, 1985 – first 7 chapters only.
2. *The Doctor, his Patient and the Illness* by Michael Balint, International Universities Press, Madison, CT, USA, 1963.
3. *Tutorials in General Practice,* by M. Meade and H. Patterson, Pitman, London, 1983.

4. *Preventative Medicine in General Practice,* by J. A. M. Gray and G. Fowler, Oxford University Press, 1983.
5. *Continuing Care: The Management of Chronic Disease,* edited by J. Hasler and T. Schofield, Oxford University Press, Oxford, 1984.
6. *Common Dilemmas in Family Medicine,* edited by John Fry, Kluwer Academic Publishers, Norwell, MA, USA, 1983.
7. *Games People Play* by Eric Berne, Ballantine Books, New York, USA, 1978.
8. *Disease Data Book* by J. Fry, G. Sandler and D. Books, Kluwer Academic Publishers, Norwell, MA, USA, 1986.

Other sources that you may find helpful include:

1. Handbook of Contraceptive Practice, DHSS, London, 1984.
2. *Basic Developmental Screening of 0–4 Years,* 3rd edn, by R. Illingworth, C. V. Mosby, St. Louis, MO, USA, 1982.
3. *Medical Aspects of Fitness to Drive,* HMSO, London, 1985.
4. *The General Practitioner's Yearbook* (Winthrop Pharmaceuticals).
5. *Medicine International* issues covering psychiatric disorders.
6. *Notes for the MRCGP,* K. T. Palmer, Blackwell Scientific, Oxford, 1988.

For self-testing the RCGP can provide past MEQ and PTQ papers (no answers available however).